MIND
GAMES

ALZHEIMER'S SOCIETY

MIND GAMES

Over 150 Puzzles to Boost Your Memory and Train Your Brain

DR TIM BEANLAND

With original puzzles by
Dr Gareth Moore

PENGUIN BOOKS

PENGUIN BOOKS

UK | USA | Canada | Ireland | Australia
India | New Zealand | South Africa

Penguin Books is part of the Penguin Random House group of companies
whose addresses can be found at global.penguinrandomhouse.com

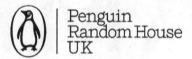

First published in Penguin Books 2023
002

Text design by Dan Prescott
Typeset in 11.5/16pt Plantin MT Pro by Jouve (UK), Milton Keynes
Printed and bound in Great Britain by Clays Ltd, Elcograf S.p.A.

The authorised representative in the EEA is Penguin Random House Ireland,
Morrison Chambers, 32 Nassau Street, Dublin D02 YH68

A CIP catalogue record for this book is available from the British Library

ISBN: 978–1–529–90167–2

www.greenpenguin.co.uk

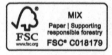

MIX
Paper | Supporting
responsible forestry
FSC® C018179

Penguin Random House is committed to a
sustainable future for our business, our readers
and our planet. This book is made from Forest
Stewardship Council® certified paper.

In memory of my mother,
Nancy Beanland
(1932–2015)

Any man could, if he were so inclined,
be the sculptor of his own brain.

Santiago Ramón y Cajal
(1852–1934), neuroscientist

If we examine the different degrees of activity of the
cerebral organs, it is necessary to consider not only
their size and organic constitution, but also the
exercise every faculty has undergone.

Johann Gaspar Spurzheim
(1776–1832), phrenologist

Your mind needs exercise just as much as your body does.
That's why I think of jogging every day.

Anon

Contents

Preface

So-called senior moments *really* annoy me. Forgetting the name of a colleague, hoping they've put their moniker in the Zoom profile. Getting to the checkout and not being able to recall your PIN even though you've used the card a hundred times. Putting your mobile down and having to ask someone to call you so you can find it again. (It is *always* in the same place in the bathroom. Why can't I just remember?)

It's not just that the phrase seems to trigger the earworm that is 'Magic Moments' in my mind. It's more how frustrating these moments are, and that sense of, 'If this now, what next?'

Such signs of 'greying' of the grey matter may be annoying. But they are not inevitable. We can all stay sharp for longer, with just a little effort. Part of that effort is about clean living: physical exercise, a healthy diet, and so on. But this book is about something else – think of it as *mental* push-ups. What do I mean? Simply that the brain is like any other muscle: to keep it trim, you've got to get to the gym. Such brain workouts can include time spent enjoying puzzles: fun *and* good for you!

As well as warding off those everyday lapses, brain workouts like regular puzzling will also help keep at bay what is now the most-feared health condition among over fifties: dementia, whether that be Alzheimer's disease, vascular dementia, or other, less common forms. In our ageing society, dementia has become one of the leading causes of death. Whatever shape it takes, dementia is a life-changing diagnosis, which is often lived with incredible courage. But currently without a cure.

Mention of the 'D word' leads me on to what Hollywood would call the 'origin story' for *Mind Games*. Of course I want you to enjoy the puzzles, stay sharp, and not get dementia. But beyond that, just by buying the book you've already changed someone's life. Every purchase of *Mind Games* is helping to fund Alzheimer's Society, the UK's leading dementia charity. Your support means we can continue to help those living with dementia now, and offer hope for better treatments and even a cure in the future.

Funding care and finding a cure for dementia have never been more needed. I know this, as I'm sure will many of you, from personal experience. My own mother Nancy lived with dementia, most of the time pretty well. In her memory and on behalf of everyone living with dementia, thank you.

Tim Beanland
Winchester, Hampshire

May 2023

Introduction

We are living on Puzzle Planet. Just look around. A woman
excitedly scribbles in the answer to 7 down as the bus lurches
along. Two old friends sit absorbed in a jigsaw, their ease with
each other in the silence so eloquent. A teenager with a Rubik's
cube showboats to a would-be girlfriend. And a student plays
Wordle, or Worldle, or Sudoku, on his phone – anything to
avoid having to start *that* essay. Puzzles are everywhere.

We enjoy puzzles partly because they're different from the
challenges of everyday life – 'If we invite Chris, what about
Sunita?' – because we know there is a neat and tidy answer
waiting to be discovered, rather than a fudgy compromise.

Lack of a tidy solution makes for an unhappy puzzler. Lewis
Carroll has the Mad Hatter famously tease, 'Why is a raven like
a writing-desk?', but then give no answer. Carroll's Victorian
readers pestered him so much that he was forced to retro-fit
what was for him a pretty weak solution: 'Because it can
produce a few notes'. Rest assured that all the puzzles in
Mind Games come with tidy answers.

The power of puzzles

Something that has become apparent only very late in the long history of puzzles is how they might help to solve one of the biggest challenges society faces. For Puzzle Planet is now a Greying Globe. Life expectancy in the UK has historically, since the mid-nineteenth century, risen by three months *every year*. Reason to celebrate, but it comes at a price. More of us will also live to see the effects of brain ageing – those moments when we get a bit muddled or forget someone's name. And on Greying Globe, more of us risk developing diseases closely linked to ageing, including such devastating conditions as dementia.

At Alzheimer's Society, we see both sides of this. It's quite common for people who are actually ageing healthily to sense changes and worry that they are getting dementia. Conversely, a fair few people who really do have Alzheimer's disease lose insight and think they're actually fine.

But neither senior moments nor dementia are *inevitable* consequences of ageing. We can all stack the odds a bit more in our favour. What has become clear over the past thirty-five years is how much we can act to reduce our own risk of losing mental sharpness as we age and lower our chances of getting dementia. We shall see that this is a story of two halves. One half is firmly focused on bodily wellbeing: a lifestyle of physical exercise, healthy eating, good sleep, and consuming toxins like alcohol only in moderation (if at all). 'What's good for the heart is good for the head,' we will learn to chant.

The other half of our story is – thankfully – less puritanical. It is about cognitive stimulation, those mental push-ups, and that is where the puzzles come in. As we will learn, regular workouts of the grey matter can help you stay sharp as you get older. As if that were not enough, mental stimulation like this also helps to reduce your chances of developing dreaded diseases like Alzheimer's. Anything to stack the odds a bit more in our favour is surely worth having.

So, this book is where Puzzle Planet and Greying Globe overlap. Where Sudoku meets senior moments, anagrams meet Alzheimer's. *Mind Games* starts with some reflections on our ageing society, what is happening and attitudes towards it. I argue that *ageing well* is a possibility – even something we should all aspire to. Ageing well leads us into what happens to our brains as we get older, in health and in age-related diseases such as stroke and Alzheimer's. We'll see how some loss in thinking speed, attention, and memory can come with age, but also how you can fight back against this. And how, like a good wine, some functions of our brain improve with the years.

Armed with some background, you're then into the puzzles. These are arranged by type (based on words, pictures, numbers, and so on) so that you are exercising different parts of your brain. Variety is the spice of brain health! The puzzles get harder as you go through them, so you're really challenging that grey matter. When it comes to your brain, it really is a case of 'Use it or lose it'. I've given you a suggested puzzle workout routine to get the most out of them.

But how does this brain workout really keep you sharp and help stave off dementia? That's a story about brain resilience, the brain's way of absorbing a lot of disease without buckling to symptoms. And it's a story with some fascinating characters. Roman Catholic nuns, London taxi drivers, people speaking two languages, and musicians all have tales to tell about how the brain benefits from being challenged.

You then get another chapter of puzzles to tease you, including some that will really exercise the grey matter.

Finally, we look at neuroplasticity, a really hot topic in brain science. That sounds a bit geeky, but without it none of the above would be possible. Puzzles can change your brain only because it is so malleable. Regularly doing puzzles taps into this lifelong plasticity to help us build brain resilience. And that is what is helping you to stay sharp and free from dementia. I've also thrown in some occasional trivia as a bonus: is 'grey matter' really grey, and – if so – why? Can fish count? A cruciverbalist is someone who . . . ? Read on to find out.

I hope that knowing a bit more about what's going on as you do the puzzles, and the benefits that solving them brings, is interesting. Knowing the benefits might even motivate you to keep going to find the answer. Happy puzzling!

1. 'Fade to Grey'

When Anne Robinson announced, aged seventy-seven, that she was stepping down as the ice-queen host of *Countdown*, she joked, 'Now it is time for an older woman to take the reins.'

How could someone in their late seventies or even eighties possibly host a TV game show, let alone *Countdown*, with its quickfire anagrams and mental maths? I mean they'd surely be too, well . . . old?

I'm going to tell a different story about ageing, one in which we ditch the doom and gloom for a brighter future. While there are no quick fixes or snake-oil cures, the story is more positive than you might think, and also within your grasp.

We will look at these questions:

- Are we living healthier, or just longer, than we used to?
- How ageist is the UK now – and does it matter?
- Can how you think about yourself affect how well you age?
- Could we change how we think about ageing as a society? What would the benefits be?

Living in the age of ageing

In the UK, everyone who lives to 100 still gets a congratulatory message from the monarch. During the long reign of the late Queen Elizabeth II, reaching this milestone – although still unusual – became much more common. On her accession in 1952, there were just 300 centenarians in the UK. By the end of her reign in 2022, there were more than 15,000. (The UK population rose from 50 million to 67 million over that time, so nowhere near as steeply.) It is easy to keep forgetting it, because – like the passage of time itself – things have crept up on us, but we are living in the age of ageing. Forget the cool, shiny blue of sci-fi films. The future is grey.

This shift is driven less by those centenarians – they may well be genetic outliers – and more by the long-term historical rise in average life expectancy. According to the Office for National Statistics, average lifespans in England in the past 150 years grew on average by almost three years *every decade*. Three months of extra life each year.[1]

---

1   This long-term and seemingly inexorable march of progress has been unexpectedly interrupted twice in recent years. Since 2011, life expectancy in England has continued to grow, but less quickly than it had for the previous century – the causes are hotly debated. Worse was to come. In 2020–21, the excess deaths caused by Covid-19 meant that life expectancy fell sharply, by a degree not seen since World War 2. What will happen to life expectancy now is maybe less certain than it felt in 2000.

And not just in England. A similar story of population ageing is playing out across Europe, North America, and Japan. The rest of the world is catching up fast too. What is happening in the world's wealthiest countries today will happen in the likes of Brazil, India, and China tomorrow. And in the low-income countries the day after.[2]

This rise in life expectancy has been oddly clocklike in its consistency. In the nineteenth century, better diet, hygiene, housing, and sanitation all helped to extend lives. (You might have heard of Joseph Bazalgette's sewers and John Snow's water pump.) Since the 1950s, rising life expectancy has been driven more by childhood vaccination, the introduction of the NHS, better treatments for heart disease and cancer, and fewer people smoking. Increases in average life expectancy were historically caused by saving younger lives but are now driven by older people staying alive for longer.

Reasons for this rise aside, the numbers are striking. In 1920, average life expectancy for women in England was about sixty years and for men about fifty-six. By 2020, women's life expectancy was eighty-three years and men's seventy-nine.[3]

---

2   It could actually happen faster than this chronology implies because the rate of ageing is quickening. In France, it took nearly 150 years for the over sixties to rise from accounting for 10 per cent of the population to 20 per cent. India is now set to do that in little more than two decades.

3   Women have outlived men in pretty much all countries for as long as data have been collected, probably due to a mix of biology and lifestyle. But the gap is gradually narrowing: in England it was six years in 1981 but is under four years today.

This long-term trend in rising life expectancy coincides with a halving of average fertility rates (i.e. births per woman) globally since 1950. In nearly every country, couples are having fewer children. So, on the conveyer belt of life that drives population age profiles, fewer babies are crawling on and the oldies are staying on for longer.

The implications of all this for society are dramatic. Projections in England suggest that the proportion of the population older than sixty-five will rise from 18 per cent in 2020 to 27 per cent by 2065. For over eighty-fives, the rise over this period will be even steeper, from 2.5 per cent to 6 per cent. Globally, low- and middle-income countries will see even more dramatic rises. By 2050, two-thirds of all the world's over sixties will live in low- or middle-income countries.

What we die *from* has changed dramatically too. In the 1920s and 1930s, infectious diseases and cancer were the leading causes of death. By the 1950s, heart disease became the leading cause, as tuberculosis was increasingly treated with new antibiotics.

Covid-19 reminded us not to become complacent about infection, and flu and pneumonia are usually still among the most common causes of death in the UK. But the leading cause of death for ten years in the UK has as often as not been dementias, such as Alzheimer's disease. You might know that Alzheimer's is caused by brain disease but not have thought of dementia as a terminal condition. But it is life-limiting: if a person gets dementia, they are not going to be around as long, everything else being equal, as if they hadn't got it.

Why is dementia now such a big killer? Stroke and heart disease used to head the list but in the past twenty years these conditions are killing far fewer people, largely because of better medical treatments. But dementia has – unique among the top ten killers in the UK – no drug treatment to prevent, cure, or slow it down. The brain has with good reason, if little respect for anatomy, been called the Achilles heel of ageing. So, as more people survive heart disease and stroke, they live long enough for some to get (and then die from) dementia in unprecedented numbers.

Lifespan versus healthspan

Alongside our tale of *total* life expectancy is a story about *healthy* life expectancy. Put simply, that is the time you live free from poor health, which is sometimes called 'healthspan'.

As lifespans have risen, have healthspans followed suit? The picture is a bit messy but, in the fifteen years to 2020, total healthspan has fallen for both men and women. On average in the UK, more than 20 per cent of life is now lived with disability.

Could we reduce those years spent in poor health, so that healthspan grows as a proportion of lifespan? The jargon for this squeezing of poor health into fewer years is 'compression of morbidity'. ('Morbus' is the Latin word for 'disease'.) This is already the experience of some people with dementia: they live longer free from dementia, then develop it later in life and live with it for a shorter time.

So, where does this leave us? The long-term rise in life expectancy has been hailed as the greatest achievement of the past century. It will shape our lives in ways we are only just

starting to realise. When the basic UK state pension was
introduced in 1948, life for a lot of people followed a fairly
predictable pattern: you worked (probably in one job or career)
and if you got to retirement age you put your feet up for a few
years at most. And then you were done. In contrast, when
someone reaches state pension age in the UK today – itself a
moving target as time goes by – they can expect to live another
sixteen years. That's more than a fifth of our lives.

Those extra years certainly offer a huge potential opportunity,
especially if more of them could be enjoyed in good health and
happiness. How would you want to live them? What if everyone
stayed active and engaged, healthy in mind and body? How
about travelling, learning a new language or maybe – after a
well-earned break – training for a new career?

This opportunity is the broad canvas on which *Mind Games* is
painted. You will, I hope, get deeply engaged in the puzzles. But,
while there, just occasionally switch your perspective – a bit like
flipping a Necker cube[4] – back to this broader picture. Shift
from the *Games* to the *Mind* if you like, and by extension to
your brain and its future. Where do you want to take it?

Such musing aside, our ageing society undeniably also poses
huge challenges. What does it mean – for all of us – to live in a
world increasingly made up of older people? With those falling
birth rates, will there be enough future taxpayers to fund health

---

4   The Necker cube is an optical illusion of a cube drawn as a wireframe
    in three dimensions. Most people tend to interpret it as being oriented
    one way, but with a little mental effort they are able to 'flip' it to a
    different view. Google it and try yourself.

and social care, let alone workers to provide support for older people who might need it? What about the looming pensions crisis? It's easy to see this as a tale that sets generation against generation, young against old.

Where do you stand on all this? That grey future is a train barrelling inexorably towards us all. Do you jump aboard for the ride or stand aside and let it whoosh by?

Your answer will depend partly on how you think about older people. It may well depend on how old you are, or even how old you *feel*. Anne Robinson's salvo on leaving *Countdown* set out the challenge: 'I hope, too, I've encouraged TV bosses to realise that not all women at the wrong end of their seventies are in care homes playing bingo and watching conjuring tricks.' But is it just TV bosses who (allegedly) think that? Let's look at attitudes to ageing.

Thinking differently about ageing

What comes to mind when you think of an old person? It might be a very positive picture, but if your mental image is of someone who is frail, has lost the plot a bit, and needs help, you're not alone. Such a bleak take on ageing has a distinguished pedigree, captured most famously by Shakespeare in *As You Like It*:

> *Last scene of all,*
> *That ends this strange eventful history,*
> *Is second childishness and mere oblivion;*
> *Sans teeth, sans eyes, sans taste, sans everything.*

How we all think about older people and ageing will affect what
we do about our changing society, and what we'll do ourselves
as we age. Let's look at some more recent evidence.

A 2021 report by the Centre for Ageing Better charity
summarised public attitudes towards ageing in England. What
they call the 'dominant view' is pretty bleak. That attitude sees
ageing as an inevitable decline: all those aches and pains, and
loss of vision, hearing, strength, and mental sharpness – and
worse. In this pessimistic view, ageing leads only to dependency
and death, which means that older people are all frail,
vulnerable, and in need of support. A burden. Getting old,
according to this view, is something that should be feared rather
than embraced.

Drill down into the survey data and attitudes vary according to
the age of who you ask. People aged fifty to sixty-nine were the
most negative overall about ageing – perhaps because they are
the 'sandwich generation', supporting children and elderly
parents while still having to work. In contrast, the over seventies
were the most positive about ageing. Many of them spoke of
having more time and a sense of freedom. The survey doesn't
say, but you can easily imagine how someone's health might
colour this view, and there is evidence of that elsewhere. Many
people begin to feel 'old inside' because of long-term or
repeated poor health, or when disability begins to restrict daily
life. But even there we vary.

In the Centre for Ageing Better survey, people aged eighteen to
thirty-four were most likely to see older age as a time of frailty
and dependency. Separate studies show that ageism is much
less common among young people who have actually spent time

with older people.[5] So, a pessimistic view of ageing seems to be held more by those yet to experience later life. That kind of makes sense. In Chapter 3 we look in detail at ageing and the brain. We'll see that the reality of how our minds age is much more positive than most people think. A lot of things improve as the years go by.

Why do attitudes to ageing matter, both in general and when we think about brain health as we age? In lots of different ways, ageism prevents people from ageing well and even leads to faster loss of mental and physical abilities, and an earlier death.

In short, if we think in an ageist way (in stereotypes), it can affect how we feel (prejudice) and hence how we behave (discrimination). Such discrimination might mean that an older person isn't considered for a job, is unfairly denied the healthcare that a younger person might get, becomes socially isolated or depressed, is treated like a child in a care home ('second childishness'), or is portrayed negatively in the media. At a time of greater awareness of the need to fight discrimination in all its forms, some have called ageism 'the last socially acceptable prejudice'.[6] It's well documented that different forms of discrimination – racism, sexism, ageism, and so on – overlap and reinforce each other. These interactions are increasingly

---

5   Spending time with older relatives has become less common in the UK, thanks to our long-distance families and the way we look after so many more of our oldest in care homes.

6   'Ageism is one of the last socially acceptable prejudices. Psychologists are working to change that' by Kirsten Weir, *Monitor on Psychology* (March 2023).

discussed under the framework of 'intersectionality', although definitions of that are evolving, contextual, and contested. Hollywood often excludes older women from the script, but manages to find roles for older men.

I've been looking mainly at data for England, but these kinds of attitudes cross national boundaries. The United Nations Decade of Healthy Ageing (2021–2030) lists combatting ageism as one of its four areas for action.

It's fairly easy to imagine how someone might be ageist towards another person. What is less obvious is how we might hold stereotyped attitudes towards our *own* age – self-directed ageism. If you've ever thought, 'I'd like to enrol on that language course or try that exercise class, but I'm too old to learn something new,' you've acted with self-directed ageism.

This kind of prophecy can easily become self-fulfilling. This is a risk for many people who enter a settled mid-life, but it can happen at any age. We tell ourselves we're too old to try something new, so we don't. The risk is that we lose our self-confidence to try new things and get into a habit of safe routines. We go to the same places, we see the same people, we do the same things. It's called a comfort zone for a reason. And it's not somewhere to settle if you want to help your body or brain to age well.

Or think about how your choices influence those around you. Have you ever nearly bought a slightly trendier outfit, for example, which you really fancied – but didn't? A little voice said, 'It's too young for you,' so you went for a safer option. Choices like that certainly affect how other people view us. If others look at our choices and think they're a bit old, they're more likely to treat us as old. Ageism is almost infectious. You can see how all this might spiral down.

But spirals go up as well as down. Circles can be virtuous as well as vicious. Another finding from the Centre for Ageing Better survey was that people older than fifty often felt 'young inside' and sometimes acted younger than their 'real' age – though 'acting your age' as a concept has more than a whiff of self-directed ageism. That 'acted' is vital in all this. By *doing* things, especially things that are new or challenging, we expose our brains to experiences that allow us to change and grow. We'll learn a lot more about how our brains respond to variety, novelty, and challenge – including puzzles – later. Your amazing brain retains a lifelong ability to reinvent itself over and over. Stimulating it does just that, forging new neural networks, and making your grey matter stronger and more resilient.

So, to summarise, society is ageing more quickly than attitudes seem to be adjusting to that fact. Older people themselves tend to see old age more positively, especially if they retain reasonable health. They often report a renewed sense of purpose and wellbeing, with greater emotional stability. Why can't we all take a lead from older people and start thinking differently about ageing? Let's see where that would lead us.

Healthy ageing

What is the alternative to the pessimistic view of ageing as an inevitable decline, from 'mere oblivion' to death? It's a reframing in which, rather than being seen as frail and dependent, older people still lead active and engaged lives. In short, healthy ageing.

This more positive view sees ageing as something to accept and adapt to rather than defy. But accepting ageing doesn't mean being defeatist about it. What if instead we choose to embrace the good things about later life – freedom to make choices on your own terms, more time for new hobbies or travel, perhaps being an active grandparent – rather than continuously chasing after youth? What if we used our wealth of experience to reframe the events that life will still throw our way as opportunities to learn?

Life has followed a linear path for generations: birth, education, work, retirement, death. But with healthy ageing, we can break free from that. Why not a career break to travel or learn new skills, followed by trying out a different career?

A healthy-ageing agenda like this has been brewing quietly for a while – perhaps too quietly judging from public opinions in that survey. Clearly a lot of people are still with the Bard on this. I've already summarised the changes in how we think about getting older behind this agenda. Medically, ageing well means that healthy life expectancy would be extended, and the time spent in poor health, disability or dependency would be squashed into a shorter period at the end of life. (To think we can avoid *any* such period is at the moment pure sci-fi.[7]) That extended healthspan would mean more people would remain sharp as

---

7   For an optimistic recent take on a 'cure for ageing' see Andrew Steele's *Ageless: The New Science of Getting Older Without Getting Old* (Bloomsbury, 2020).

they aged, keeping mentally active and engaged in life. It would also mean fewer people developing dementia, or getting it much later in life and living with it for less time.

That compression of morbidity would benefit individuals and also stretched health and social care systems, because so much effort goes into caring for older people in hospital and care homes towards the end of their lives.

In this more positive view of ageing, healthier and happier older people would actively participate in, and contribute to, society much more than at present. For that contribution, whether it be via paid work, volunteering or caring for grandchildren, older people have a wealth of experience and skills to draw on, a broader perspective on life, and a greater emotional resilience. They have, after all, done a fair bit of living.

Longer lives would then become not a burden but an opportunity – for society, for the economy, for families, and for individuals.

The dominant, ageist view is sometimes characterised as 'Ageing is about old people'. Our more positive view of active healthy ageing has a different slogan: 'Ageing is a lifelong process.' This may seem counter-intuitive, but it conveys that ageing starts at birth and is an extended, ongoing process. Ageing is driven by multiple interactions: between our biology and psychology, but much more so by the opportunities we get and the choices we make, as well as by wider social, systemic and environmental factors. These forces that affect how we age operate *throughout* our lives, from birth to death. Thus, this view of ageing is called a 'life-course' approach.

In this new view, different stages of life bring different experiences, opportunities, and challenges, but older age is not different in kind from any other life stage. Old age is much more a continuation of the rest of life than it is different. The life-course approach to ageing has some big implications. One is that, although it's never too late to start looking after yourself, to live a healthy older age you should start young if you can.

We touched on some examples of how to promote healthy ageing earlier when we discussed self-directed ageism. In a nutshell, the keys to ageing well are: be an optimist (if you can), stay engaged and curious about life, keep learning and challenging yourself with new things, and, above all, *be active*. Keep moving, keep meeting people, keep learning, keep mentally stimulated – and that includes puzzling!

The other keys to ageing well will be familiar if you've read any of the books on the 'How to live a longer, healthier life' shelf. The authors here are people like Dr Rangan Chatterjee with his 'four pillars' of relaxation, diet, physical exercise, and sleep. I summarise some of this in Appendix 2, but with a focus on brain health rather than on overall health. There are, as we'll see, some big overlaps between brain health and overall health, and between healthy brain ageing and healthy bodily ageing.

If you follow all this advice – and do all the puzzles – you will at the same time be helping your heart, blood vessels, lungs, and liver as well as your grey matter. In other words, you should live longer and happier to make the most of that healthier head. Let's look at its contents next.

2. Brain basics

Before you get into the puzzles, it's helpful to know a bit about your grey matter, so you can understand how it is affected by ageing and what exactly the puzzles are exercising. So, how do your brain and its nerve cells work?

'The brain is a world consisting of a number of unexplored continents and great stretches of unknown territory,' wrote the Nobel laureate and father of modern neuroscience, Santiago Ramón y Cajal, way back in 1906.

More than a century on, our understanding of the brain and how it works remains paradoxical. With access to so much technology, research funding, and human ingenuity, new discoveries in neuroscience flood the specialist literature and the news daily. Yet how brain activity leads to consciousness – that subjective sensation of self – remains, like Churchill's Russia, 'a riddle, wrapped in a mystery, inside an enigma'.

Since long before Ramón y Cajal, the metaphors for how we think about the brain have changed repeatedly, usually in line with the leading tech of the time. In the seventeenth century, the brain was a machine like a clock or the then-fashionable automaton. To the Victorians, the brain was first an electric battery, then a telegraph. Later it was a telephone switchboard.

Since the 1950s, we've become used to comparisons drawn from computers, coding or artificial intelligence. All of these metaphors have become strained sooner or later.

Fortunately for both of us, our needs in this chapter are much more modest than corralling consciousness or musing about metaphors. With an eye firmly on what we will need to know later, we will look at these questions:

- How do scientists study the brain?
- What is its large-scale structure?
- How does that relate to brain function?
- What are nerve cells, and how do they work?

This might feel a bit remote from the puzzles, but it will really help you to appreciate which parts of the grey matter get worked out by the different puzzles. Seatbelts on!

Studying the brain

The living human brain presents a challenge to anyone seeking to make it less of a riddle: it is firmly encased in the skull and gets distinctly unhappy if tampered with or removed. Despite this, scientists have over time found ways to breach the barriers to studying the brain.[1]

Since the nineteenth century, studies of patients with damage ('lesions') to certain parts of the brain – caused by disease,

---

1   For more about the history of neuroscience and the brain, see Matthew Cobb's *The Idea of the Brain* (Profile Books, 2021).

trauma, or surgery – have been key to revealing how the brain works.

An early and now famous case study is that of Phineas Gage, a foreman in the burgeoning but health-and-safety-light mid-nineteenth century US rail network. In 1848, while cutting a railroad bed in Vermont, Gage was packing explosive powder into a hole with a tamping iron. The powder went off unexpectedly and Gage's close encounter of the second kind with the forty-inch-long iron saw it propelled at speed up through his left cheek and out through the front of his skull. The rod is reported as landing several dozen feet away. Gage was blinded in his left eye but by some miracle survived, although his personality did not: he became withdrawn and impulsive. He indulged 'at times in the grossest profanity'.

The standard story that such case studies tell us is simple, probably too simple. If a lesion in part of the brain causes loss of an ability (for Gage, self-control) then that ability must reside in – or be 'localised' to – the damaged area (the front part of the brain). This idea of 'localisation' of brain function is helpful, but it will take us only so far.

Fast forward nearly a century to the 1930s and electroencephalography (EEG) is king: think of those photos of people sitting bemusedly with a hatful of electrodes dotted over their scalps. EEG relies on the surprising fact that a lot of brain activity, the sum of millions of nerve cells firing, can be picked up on the skull. Different kinds of activity – sleeping, resting, solving problems and puzzles – all cause brain waves with signature frequencies. But EEG is used a lot less now that brain scans are here. It's cheap and portable, but EEG can't tell where in the brain the signal is coming from.

For more than fifty years, techniques that show the structure or workings of the living human brain – in health and disease – have opened up whole new vistas of medicine and research. Such imaging technology includes computed tomography (CT), in which the body is X-rayed in slices – like slicing a Battenberg cake, but with much more detail and a lot less marzipan. Head CT provides a static picture of the structure of brain tissue.

Using radio waves and a powerful magnet rather than X-rays, magnetic resonance imaging (MRI) came a few years after CT. MRI also produces a black-and-white image of the anatomy of the brain in slices, hence the term 'structural MRI', but MRI scans usually show a lot more detail than CT scans.

The explosion of knowledge about the brain in recent years has come from not structural but 'functional' MRI. As the name suggests, functional MRI looks at brain activity rather than anatomy. The brain uses a lot of oxygen, even more when it's busy. Functional MRI detects the amount of oxygenated blood flowing into certain parts of the brain, which is a measure of how active the nerve cells in that region are. The clever part is that functional MRI can measure this while a person is doing a task. They could be looking at pictures, being asked to imagine saying the word 'pencil' or – I kid you not – having an orgasm. In each case, different regions of the brain are active or said to 'light up'.

There is a lot of technical wizardry needed behind the scenes to create such MRI scans, but if you see a picture of the brain with regions magically lit up in different colours, there's a good chance it will be a functional scan.

If you could see your brain like this when you were doing the puzzles, there might be lights flashing on and off in quick succession almost everywhere.

Brain structure and function

What have we learned from all that studying? A lot. The human brain at just three pounds (1.3–1.4 kg) in weight is the most complicated structure we know. Thankfully a simple diagram like figure 1 will provide enough detail to start with. We're interested mainly in the largest part of the brain, which is called the cerebrum. That is home to the higher brain functions that you will use to do the puzzles.

Most of what you can see in a whole brain is cerebral cortex, a layer of nerve cells a few millimetres thick at the surface of the cerebrum. The cortex (Latin for 'bark') is a sheet of tissue that covers almost the whole brain and is intricately folded to increase its surface area. Some of the grooves in the cortex are deep enough to carve out four lobes, as shown in figure 1. The cerebrum is also divided from back to front into two mirrored halves (left and right cerebral hemispheres), with four lobes in each half.

It is helpful to assign distinct roles to each of the brain's lobes, as in figure 1. For example, parts of the frontal lobe are 'in charge of' planning, and setting goals and tasks ('executive function', like a chief exec) whereas the occipital lobe focuses on the initial processing of signals from the eyes (a key step in vision).

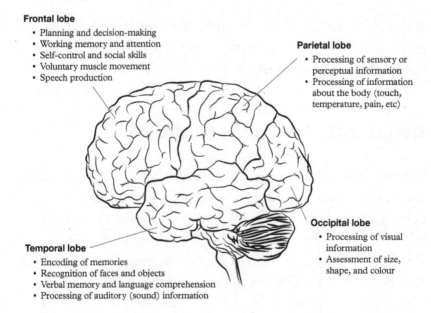

Frontal lobe
- Planning and decision-making
- Working memory and attention
- Self-control and social skills
- Voluntary muscle movement
- Speech production

Parietal lobe
- Processing of sensory or perceptual information
- Processing of information about the body (touch, temperature, pain, etc)

Occipital lobe
- Processing of visual information
- Assessment of size, shape, and colour

Temporal lobe
- Encoding of memories
- Recognition of faces and objects
- Verbal memory and language comprehension
- Processing of auditory (sound) information

Figure 1: The left side of the human brain showing the four lobes of the cerebral cortex, with some of their main functions

There are many more structures below the surface cortex that we won't discuss much, but one that we definitely will is the hippocampus (from the Greek for 'seahorse', from its shape). The hippocampus is a small structure that sits inside each temporal lobe, so it's also paired: two hippocampi. The hippocampus is the brain structure most closely linked to learning and forming new memories. It gets damaged early on in Alzheimer's, which is why memory loss is the signature symptom of that disease.

The idea that roles can be assigned to discrete regions of the cortex – cerebral localisation – dates back to the mid-nineteenth century, when those lesion studies proved so influential. But we now know, partly from functional MRI scans, that the brain's higher functions – vision, language, long-term memory, solving puzzles – require many different parts to work together. Specialised regions deliver cognitive functions[2] only by being connected into a series of pathways or a network. A pathway can involve parts of several lobes and often deeper parts of the brain too, below the cortex. A network typically weaves back and forth across the brain, like a cat's cradle. This completely debunks the myth that you only use 10 per cent of your brain at once.

And now a key point about pathways or networks for you to file away: those that are used more get stronger – a clear example of 'Use it or lose it'. Making stronger connections like this is part of healthy brain ageing.

Another 'side' to cerebral localisation is the brain's two hemispheres, left and right. You might have read that these do different things, or even have different characters. The brain's left side is meant to be analytical, mathematical and logical whereas the right is all about bringing information together and being creative or artistic – you can almost predict their taste in clothes. But this view is now largely out of fashion because most brain tasks involve both hemispheres. The main exception is

---

2   The brain's highest-level tasks (cognitive function) are usually divided into a handful of 'domains', including learning and memory, language, and executive function. You will come across these soon when you do the puzzles.

language, which *is* very much left-sided.[3] 'Visuospatial relations', which include how we perceive three dimensions and navigate around our environment, are also heavily lateralised, this time to the right side of the brain.

Given that most brain tasks use both hemispheres, it is fortunate that the two halves are connected by a bundle of more than 200 million nerve fibres. This corpus callosum ('tough body') is there to carry signals between the two hemispheres. It is the largest white-matter structure in the brain. (See below for more about white matter.)

Nerve cells and how they work

Neurons or nerve cells are the most important cells in the brain. There are other cells called glial[4] cells, which have a vital 'supporting actor' role, but the neurons get top billing. A healthy adult brain has on average about 86 billion of them. Brain activity – thought, talk, touch – is all based on electrical and chemical signals flowing between nerve cells connected into neural networks.

The complexity of those networks is mind-blowing. Each of the 86 billion adult nerve cells connects with up to 10,000–15,000

---

3   Language is lateralised to the left side of the brain in more than 90 per cent of right-handed people and in 75 per cent of left-handers. So, only a small minority of people have language lateralised to the right side of their brain.

4   Their name comes from the Greek for 'glue', reflecting a now-discarded idea that glia somehow hold (glue) neurons in place.

other neurons, so the total number of connections in the cortex is many tens of trillions.[5]

How does a nerve cell work? Each neuron (figure 2) has a roundish cell body that houses its nucleus, where most of its DNA is stored. The neuron also contains many mitochondria – the 'powerhouses' of the cell. These use oxygen to extract energy from the brain's fuel of sugar and so hold a small voltage (70 millivolts) across the nerve cell's outer membrane. When a neuron fires or spikes, that voltage suddenly collapses – like a Jenga tower falling down – and that appears as an electrical signal pulsing along the cell.

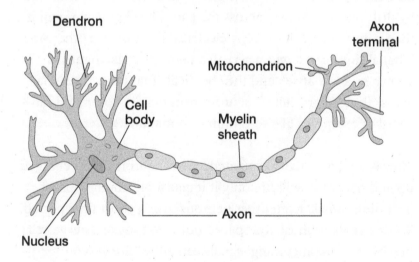

Figure 2: Structure of a neuron

---

5   A trillion is a thousand billion or one followed by twelve zeros (1,000,000,000,000). The number of connections (synapses) in the healthy adult brain cortex is about 100,000,000,000,000.

Tens of thousands of branch-like outgrowths called dendrites or
dendrons (both mean 'tree'), themselves with smaller branches
called spines, bring electrical signals *into* the cell body. Carrying
signals *away* from the cell body is a long, thin axon. This
branches at the end (the axon terminal) to reach out to other
nerve cells.

To build up pathways, the axon terminals of one nerve cell
connect with the dendritic spines or cell body of another nerve
cell. Where two neurons meet like this there is a narrow gap
across which an electrical signal cannot pass. Instead, the
current zipping along the axon is temporarily converted from
an electrical into a chemical signal, which carries the message
by drifting more slowly across the gap. The chemical signal is
then converted back to zippy electrical form on the other side.
That all-important gap where two neurons shake hands is
known as a 'synapse', and the chemicals that ferry the signal
across the gap are called 'neurotransmitters'. (You might have
heard of examples like serotonin or dopamine.)

How is all that activity regulated? Each neuron sits all charged
up and ready but will fire only if it gets a big enough jolt of
incoming signals from other neurons over a short time period.
Weak signals or those too spaced out won't make a nerve cell
fire. Now, those incoming signals can either fire (excite) or
dampen down (inhibit) the neuron, depending on the
neurotransmitter. So, to fire, the neuron needs to tally up inputs
from the thousands of other neurons it's connected to over a
short timeframe and then fire – or not: it's all or nothing. The
neuron is connected to thousands of other downstream
neurons, so when it fires it's sending signals on to all of
them too.

Incidentally, the structure of each nerve cell is what gives the whole brain its colours. The grey matter, which is mainly in the few millimetres of wrinkled cortex, is a pinky-grey because all the nerve cell bodies are there.[6] Beneath that and filling much of the brain volume is the white matter. This is made up of bundles of axons that connect distant areas of the brain like thick electricity cables. Each axon has an insulating sheath like the plastic coating on a wire, to help it carry its signal quickly without interference. The axon coat is made from a fatty substance called myelin and is formed as special glial cells wrap around the axon. Myelin is what gives white matter its colour.

So, that's some brain basics, presented in a static state. For the rest of the book we'll be looking at *changes* to the brain: first what happens with ageing and disease, and then what happens when you do the puzzles. Prepare to nurture those networks and pump those pathways!

---

6   When I write about 'giving the grey matter a workout' (or similar), I
    am using 'grey matter' figuratively, as a metaphor for the mind or
    intellect. I do also use 'grey matter' in a literal sense to contrast with
    'white matter'. The brain needs both grey and white matter to be
    healthy if it is to work at its best.

3. In sickness and in health

Brain–liver–heart. That might sound like a version of rock–paper–scissors played in an abattoir. But think for a moment about those three organs. We can't live without them, and we've all got just one of each.

Those facts mean that we ought to look after these organs carefully. I suspect you know how to look after your heart and maybe your liver a bit ('Cheers!'). But the brain, the organ that makes you 'you' and the one that you can't get a transplant for. How do you keep that in good trim?

This chapter looks at brain health, how it changes as we age, and what happens when the brain gets diseased. I will answer these questions:

- What do we mean by 'brain health'?
- Should we expect to lose our mental faculties a bit as we get older?
- What are the changes in the ageing brain behind all this?
- What causes stroke and dementia, the brain diseases most closely linked to ageing?
- What can we do to delay or prevent stroke and dementia?

The good news is that keeping your mind active partly answers the last question. So, whether you're already doing puzzles or just starting to pick them up, your brain will be thanking you for that. Let's find out why.

What is 'brain health'?

Good brain health is as much a part of healthy ageing as good heart or joint health are. You could make a strong case that brain health is the most important aspect of healthy ageing, if only because dementia caused by brain disease is among the leading causes of death in the UK.

But it turns out that brain health means different things to different people. It's worth spelling this out, because it highlights some key ideas that we will need later in the book.

A practising doctor – such as a neurologist – will think of brain health mainly in *clinical* terms. To them, good brain health would mean none of the signs or symptoms of brain diseases such as would be caused by dementia, stroke, infection, tumours, and so on.

A pathologist would take a different view. With a brain in front of them to slice and dice, stain and view under a microscope, they are looking for damage to brain tissues and cells. Diseases such as Alzheimer's and stroke cause changes in the brain that are easily visible under the microscope and often to the (trained) naked eye. *Pathological* brain health refers to a lack of significant signs of disease in the anatomised (literally, 'cut up') brain.

Finally, an occupational therapist, who supports people when they face challenges with everyday tasks, would take a pragmatic or *functional* view of brain health. Good brain health here would mean being able to get on with work, daily tasks, hobbies, and socialising in our normal environment.

You might reasonably expect that a person's brain health – good or bad – would be the same by all three definitions. But that is the case less often than you might think. As we will see, some people have good functional brain health but their grey matter turns out to be pathologically far from healthy.

What happens to brain health as we age?

What does normal brain ageing, in the absence of disease, look like?

That 2021 Centre for Ageing Better survey that we delved into before asked whether we should *expect* everyone to 'deteriorate physically and cognitively (i.e. their mental function)' when they get to old age. Nearly half of people questioned said they did.

That fraction is strikingly close to one from a 2022 Alzheimer's Society survey. In that, more than 40 per cent of people thought that significant memory loss – bad enough to potentially be dementia – was normal as people get older. (They're wrong.)

So, what really happens to our faculties as we age, so-called normal age-related cognitive decline? The short answer is that some of the brain's functions take a hit as the years pass, but not all start to deteriorate at the same age or worsen at the same rate. And a lot of things don't get worse: for some really useful functions, the brain gets better as we age. And our emotions tend to get more stable too. This is a far more optimistic picture than nearly half of us think.

Cognition, remember, is all the higher mental functions that make us human. It provides the *sapiens* ('wise' or 'knowing') to our *Homo* ('man'). Cognition includes memory, attention, language, perception, decision-making, and more. What happens to all these as we get older?

Let's get the bad news over with first. People vary a lot, but the brain's processing speed peaks as early as our thirties on average, before declining steadily. As the name suggests, processing speed describes how quickly someone can take in information, weigh it up, and then decide on a response: 'Do I have time to nip out of in front of that oncoming car, or should I wait?' Slower processing speed lengthens physical reaction times – like braking – as well as mental decisions.

Our ability to stay focused on a task – various types of attention – also falls with age. The result is that older people can be more easily distracted, and are particularly prone to be worse at switching between tasks and multitasking.[1] This means that older people might, for example, struggle more with successfully cooking a meal while listening attentively to the radio.

---

1   Multitasking in the sense of genuinely focusing on two or more tasks at once is a myth. What you're really doing is constantly switching attention between tasks. That usually makes you less, not more, efficient.

Another thing that tends to worsen from as early as thirty is working memory. That is used to manipulate information stored only briefly in your mind, such as holding someone's phone number in memory and adding it to your contacts. Working memory is, like the random-access memory (RAM) on a computer, widely used for a lot of tasks. A bit like an aged computer, older people can need more time to make decisions or reply simply because their working memory is worse.

Finally, our ability to create and recall memories that centre on ourselves tends to decline, from about age fifty or sixty, but with a lot of variation. This is known as 'episodic' memory: of events and personal experiences in life, recent or remote – what happened to us, where, and when.

How often have you gone into a room to get something (say, a book), become distracted – maybe you thought about lunch – and forgot what you went into the room for? This kind of forgetting is really common and causes a lot of middle-aged people to worry, sometimes obsessively, that they are getting Alzheimer's. What is much more likely is simply that your slightly worse working memory or attention meant you got distracted from your main task. Your working memory had stored, 'Find puzzle book', but it has limited capacity and the book idea got bumped out by, 'Ooh, tuna salad for lunch'. If you mentally retrace your steps, you will probably remember what you went in for, but it might take a moment – that's the slower processing speed.

Brain functions like these can all be affected if we are wearing the wrong glasses or a hearing aid that isn't working, if our environment is noisy or cluttered, or if we are tired, unwell, or unduly stressed. So, if someone does not respond as expected, it's possible that they have a cognitive problem, but they may simply have misheard or misread the question. In most people in most cases, these kinds of everyday mishaps are at most a mild annoyance rather than a sign of disease.

If not disease, what then causes age-related cognitive decline?

At the level of the whole brain, one of the things that happens in healthy ageing from about thirty-five onwards, and more rapidly from about age sixty, is a gradual reduction in total brain volume. This is mainly because the grey matter in the brain, including the cortex where the nerve cell bodies and dendrons live, shrinks. The cortex thins and its surface folding gets less intricate.

Another age-related change in the brain, which starts later, from about age fifty, is that the myelin sheaths around the long axons of nerve cells begin to deteriorate. This means that the different parts of the brain that the white matter connects don't talk to each other as well as they used to.

Finally, there are changes with age related to neurotransmitters, those chemicals so vital for carrying signals across synapses. The ageing brain has fewer receptors in its synapses to bind dopamine, for example.

In healthy ageing, these changes don't all affect all regions of the brain the same. Two areas are particularly vulnerable: the prefrontal cortex, with its role in planning, decision-making, and more, and the hippocampus and nearby areas, with their role in memory and learning. The prefrontal cortex is one of the last areas of the developing brain to mature. The trend towards it ageing first is sometimes referred to as 'last in, first out'.

Given the roles of these brain regions and what you now know about grey matter, white matter, and neurotransmitters, it is easy to see how the age-related changes mentioned above lead to reduced processing speed, slower decision-making, less flexibility, worse episodic memory, and so on.

What underlies these changes with ageing? One major cause of shrinking grey matter is that nerve cell bodies become less plump and the connections between neurons – the dendrons and the spines they push out – become fewer. Spines are one of the main places where synapses are formed, so their loss causes the number of synapses to fall with age. Having a less rich pattern of connections causes the brain to work less smoothly.

What ultimately lies behind all this – the root cause of ageing – is complex and not well understood. The likely suspects include mutations and other forms of damage to DNA, accumulation of cell debris and misfolded proteins, a build-up of 'senescent' cells that no longer divide, the mitochondria working less well, and weakening of the immune system.[2]

Most of these mechanisms combine with age to cause a state of persistent low-level inflammation called 'inflammageing'. When

---

2   For a good summary of current theories of ageing, see Andrew Steele's *Ageless: The New Science of Getting Older Without Getting Old* (Bloomsbury, 2020).

we are younger and get an infection or injury, our body responds with a helpful inflammatory response that comes on rapidly and then ends when it's no longer needed. This changes in later life into a harmful low-grade inflammatory response that is always on even in the absence of infection, injury or disease. Inflammageing is a hot topic because it may underpin a lot of conditions linked to ageing, including cardiovascular disease, diabetes, and dementia.

Root causes aside, two other things that definitely don't help are that glial cells, which are needed to support neurons, start to get less effective. The brain's blood supply, so essential to feed those hungry neurons, also gets worse with age.

But one thing that we now know is *not* happening in healthy ageing is significant loss of neurons in the brain. In contrast, such loss does happen in diseases like Alzheimer's. It's the reason that such conditions are known as neurodegenerative disorders: nerve cells in the brain stop working and die in large numbers. But not in normal ageing.

So much for the bad bits. What about the good?

One thing that gets better with age is so-called 'crystallised' intelligence. As the name suggests, crystallised intelligence draws on accumulated life experience, learning, and knowledge from the past – the 'wisdom of the ages' – such as vocabulary and general knowledge (both part of semantic memory). These tend to get better from age twenty, at least into our seventies. Crystallised intelligence stands in contrast to the 'fluid' intelligence covered earlier, which is about quick and flexible processing 'in the moment'. So, older people will on average perform better than younger ones on tests that rely on general knowledge, though it may take them a little longer to come up with the answer.

Decision-making that draws on experience rather than speed is another example where extra years are a help, not a hindrance. Ageing even makes people better at extracting patterns and general trends, because of accumulated experience.

As anyone who has learned a piece of music will know, 'procedural' memories – when we have learned to do something by heart and no longer need to think about it – are not affected by ageing. Riding a bike and tying shoelaces are other common examples. (Just don't try them at the same time.)

I said earlier that learning new things may become more of a challenge as we age, but the proverbial 'old dog' struggling with all 'new tricks' is too pessimistic a picture. The terrier's teacher may just need to be more patient.

All this is about cognitive ageing, but we're not robots and how well the brain works depends a lot on emotional state too. What happens to our feelings as we age?

The good news is that ageing does, in general, lead to people becoming emotionally more stable, more resilient, and more optimistic: in a word, happier. In studies from all around the world, a graph of average happiness by age is U-shaped. Happiness is high in our youth, gradually dips to a trough at about age fifty and then takes off again, perhaps unexpectedly still rising from sixty to seventy and beyond.

All the above are generalisations, and people's mental faculties change in different ways and at different rates. Why? Your genes play a role, but they are only a small part of the story. Most of the difference comes down to some core themes that we've seen already and will come back to.

Your brain, as remarkable as it is, is still an organ. So, good brain health means looking after your general health, especially your heart. Regular physical activity, a balanced diet, sleeping well, and not smoking are all really important. It's also important to keep any health conditions that you do pick up – high blood pressure, heart disease, diabetes – under control. But healthy brain ageing is also more likely if you stay mentally and socially active, because these really do give your brain a workout. We will see later how these build up brain resilience, which can reduce the effects of cognitive ageing.

So, to summarise: your brain at fifty or sixty is – like your legs – probably not going to be as quick as it was at twenty. But a lot of what we think are signs of dreaded diseases like Alzheimer's for someone in normal health are not: they are caused by distractions, sensory losses, excess stress,[3] and so on. Your accumulated knowledge and experience of those extra years is a bonus, and you're likely to get emotionally more positive as you age.

---

3   Not all stress is bad for us. A little stress under control helps us maintain attention and learn. It's when stress becomes severe, long-term or out of our control that it damages our cognition or health.

This is reassuring, but remember it all applies to normal ageing, good brain health. What happens in people who age with poor brain health, and – crucially – what can be done about that?

Brain disease

The brain is so complicated that it's no surprise there are a zillion different ways it can go wrong. Brain disorders range from tumours to trauma, from infections to inflammation and delirium, from epilepsy and stroke to neurodegenerative diseases such as Alzheimer's and Parkinson's. And this list does not even include mental illnesses – things like anxiety, depression, schizophrenia, bipolar disorder, phobias, and eating disorders.

For our purposes, the two brain disorders that we will need to know a bit about are stroke and dementia. To focus on these is not to downplay the importance of all the other brain and mind disorders. But in exploring cognition and ageing, stroke and dementia are where the breadcrumbs lead us.

Let's follow Hansel and Gretel into the brain.

Stroke

Your brain is hungry and impatient. Hungry because of all that electrical and chemical activity it needs to support: the brain accounts for just 2 per cent of your body weight but uses 20 per cent of all the body's energy. Impatient because it needs to be constantly fuelled by the blood bringing in sugar (glucose), which it can store a bit of, and oxygen, which it can't store much of at all.

Your brain health flatlines if its supply abruptly stops, as in a stroke. Suddenly the brain is no longer getting enough blood and hence not enough oxygen. The consequences can be fatal.

Stroke is called a 'cerebrovascular' disease because it involves the blood vessels in your brain – 'cerebro' means brain (as in 'cerebrum') and 'vascular' means blood vessel. By far the most common cause of stroke is a blocked artery in the brain, which is known as an ischaemic stroke. The brain artery can get blocked when a clot develops in the large arteries of the neck, or a clot can start in the heart in people with irregular heartbeats (atrial fibrillation) – the heart doesn't empty properly, so blood pools and clots – and the clot travels to the brain.[4] Ischaemic stroke deep in the brain can also follow narrowing of the very small arteries there.

In an ischaemic stroke, brain tissue that would in health be fed by the now-blocked artery is starved of oxygen and rapidly begins to die, starting in as little as minutes and creating a patch of dead tissue called an infarct. Symptoms depend on where the damaged brain tissue is, which in turn depends on which artery was blocked, and how much tissue has been lost.

When the infarct is in the surface cortex of the brain, symptoms can include problems with speech and understanding, weakness of an arm or leg on one side, or problems with planning or

---

4   Describing stroke, as here, simply in terms of 'plumbing' or a wholly 'vascular' (blood vessel) view is now known to be incomplete. Inflammation acts soon after the blockage. As so often, it can help or hinder.

concentration (as in vascular dementia, which is discussed in more detail later).

In contrast, when a 'subcortical' stroke occurs (i.e. below the cortex), it is because very small arteries deep in the brain have become narrowed or twisted. Over time this 'small vessel disease' causes many small strokes, smaller than cortical infarcts, as well as white-matter changes. Stroke caused by worsening small vessel disease tends to cause problems with steady walking and continence. Small vessel disease is probably the major cause of vascular dementia (as discussed in the next section).

Stroke of any kind can lead to anxiety, depression and sudden swings in mood. The list of stroke symptoms feels pretty grim, but there is a ray of hope: even if parts of the brain are permanently lost to stroke, survivors may make a good level of recovery due to the brain's powers of plasticity.

What underlies stroke and what can we do to prevent it? Stroke can occur at any age but it gets increasingly likely with old age. The risk doubles every ten years from fifty-five. Age affects risk of stroke because our arteries get narrower and stiffer as we get older. Genetic, sex, and ethnic factors affect stroke risk too – men and Black or South Asian people are at increased risk, for example. But a lot of reducing your stroke risk comes down to something you can control, your lifestyle.

Age apart, the single biggest thing that increases risk of stroke is high blood pressure. The other medical conditions to try to steer clear of if you can are atherosclerosis (when arteries thicken or harden because of clogging with fatty material), high cholesterol, diabetes, and atrial fibrillation. (If you do get a condition such as diabetes, managing it well reduces your stroke risk.) It shouldn't come as a surprise, but those conditions are more likely if you don't exercise, eat badly, are overweight, drink too much or smoke. In short, to prevent stroke, you've got to look after yourself.

Dementia

Armed with what we now know about stroke, let's turn to dementia. Like stroke, there are different kinds of dementia, but we will focus on just the main ones.

Dementia is a disorder of the brain that affects cognition such that the symptoms are bad enough to get in the way of daily life. Dementia – the set of symptoms – is the result of physical diseases in the brain. It is not, contrary to what the term 'senile dementia' implies and a lot of people think, caused by normal ageing.

Dozens of different brain diseases cause dementia, but 95 per cent of cases are caused by a few main types. These common dementias all share some features. They usually start gradually with minor symptoms. They are progressive, so their effects get worse over time – often years. They shorten life expectancy and are currently incurable. But people can – with support[5] – still live well with dementia a lot of the time.

The brain changes that ultimately cause dementia probably start decades before any symptoms are noticed. For most

---

5   In the UK the leading dementia support charities are Alzheimer's Society, Dementia UK and Alzheimer Scotland. Most other countries have similar Alzheimer's associations.

people who get dementia that means changes from middle age. It's never too early to start looking after your brain.

Let's cover vascular dementia first, because it's closely related to stroke. Different forms of stroke can each cause problems with reasoning and memory, and in some cases these are severe enough to count as dementia. In small vessel disease, dementia tends to start gradually and get worse slowly. After a cortical stroke, about one in five people will have so-called 'post-stroke vascular dementia'. Dementia may then worsen in steps, with further strokes. Memory loss is a less common early symptom of vascular dementia than it is in Alzheimer's, but other symptoms – including difficulties with executive function – are shared. As with stroke, vascular dementia often makes it harder for someone to control their emotions.

'Pure' vascular dementia, in which these vascular changes are the only disease in the brain, is the second-most common form of dementia after Alzheimer's. Let's turn to that now.

Alzheimer's disease is the dementia most people have heard of. It causes about two-thirds of all dementia and we've been studying it for over 100 years. But we still don't know what really causes it.

What we see in the Alzheimer's brain over time is fairly consistent. First, levels of a key neurotransmitter called acetylcholine fall.[6] Then synapses start to be lost, before finally

---

6 Currently licensed drug treatments for Alzheimer's disease, such as donepezil, act by keeping levels of acetylcholine up. They offer some relief from symptoms, but do not treat the underlying disease.

nerve cells begin to die. This neurodegeneration typically starts in the hippocampi, which is why the signature of Alzheimer's is memory loss. To be more precise, it is the ability to form new memories that is lost, which appears as a 'rapid forgetting'. A person with Alzheimer's may ask the same question every few minutes without realising.

Over time neurodegeneration spreads from the hippocampus and nearby areas to the temporal, frontal, and parietal lobes. This is why subsequent symptoms of Alzheimer's include difficulties respectively with language, executive function, and perception in three dimensions. After several years the brain becomes lighter and – in advanced Alzheimer's disease – visibly shrunken, with a much coarser cortex. In both cases, these changes are more rapid and more severe than those seen in normal ageing. The causes are, after all, different.

Yet the root cause of this brain damage is far from an open-and-shut case. The main suspects in Alzheimer's neurodegeneration are rogue versions of two proteins: amyloid and tau. Errant fragments of β-amyloid misfold and come together, eventually forming plaques outside nerve cells. Later on tau gets chemically modified and forms filaments or 'tangles', this time inside nerve cells. The amyloid plaques and tau tangles are like cyanide pills to synapses and neurons. The spread of tau to different regions of the brain even tracks fairly closely the development of symptoms.

The idea that β-amyloid plaques are the causes of Alzheimer's disease has been around since the early 1990s and still dominates the field, such that there has been a much-needed push in the pharmaceutical industry to develop drugs that target them. That push is now, finally, beginning to bear fruit. Exciting results from trials of new drugs that successfully target β-amyloid were released in 2022 and 2023.[7] However, errant β-amyloid is not the only suggested cause of Alzheimer's in town, and a significant minority of researchers think other mechanisms matter as much or even more.

One such mechanism is cerebrovascular disease, which often has a role to play in causing Alzheimer's dementia alongside plaques and tangles. One way this could happen is by narrowing of blood vessels, reducing blood flow to the brain. As a result, less fuel is brought to the brain, and hence those hungry neurons begin to suffer. Lower blood flow also means that toxic products such as β-amyloid, which would normally get flushed out, build up. Cerebrovascular disease is particularly important when we look at risk factors for Alzheimer's.

Intriguingly, more recent evidence suggests that type 2 diabetes, which is closely linked to poor cardiovascular health and stroke, has a direct role in causing Alzheimer's via insulin resistance in the brain. Hence Alzheimer's disease has been unofficially dubbed 'type 3 diabetes'.

The links between Alzheimer's and cardiovascular disease are important but actually pretty old hat. The new kid on the block of Alzheimer's mechanisms and now vying for top billing with plaques and tangles is inflammation.

---

7 Keep an eye out for news on **alzheimers.org.uk**. These will be the first new drugs for Alzheimer's disease in twenty years, and the first treatments ever to effectively target the underlying brain pathology.

Recall how healthy ageing is linked to a state of chronic, low-level inflammation called 'inflammageing'. In Alzheimer's disease this inflammatory response is heightened and becomes more destructive. The brain has its own special immune system with cells called microglia that gobble up debris and destroy it. Microglia swarm on plaques and try to hoover up β-amyloid. But if there is too much amyloid, the microglia become persistently activated and secrete pro-inflammatory molecules. At high levels these cause loss of synapses and neurons. There is a link here with diabetes, because that too causes inflammation in the vascular systems, in the body generally and specifically in the brain.

There are other mechanisms I'm not touching on, for example related to the cell's mitochondria. If all this leaves you thinking that we don't have a good handle on what really causes Alzheimer's disease, you'd be right. The smart money is on a combination of these mechanisms acting together, possibly with some new things not yet discovered. We need more research and a lot more money to pay for it.

In addition to Alzheimer's disease, there are other less common types of dementia that have different underlying causes but the same progressive nature. They also often have overlapping symptoms, such as problems with executive function, language, and memory.

Dementia with Lewy bodies represents perhaps 15 per cent of cases of dementia, and like Alzheimer's, is caused by a misfolded protein. The culprit this time is called α-synuclein and it clumps up to form Lewy bodies. Symptoms of dementia with Lewy bodies can include memory loss but more common are hallucinations, changes in alertness, really disturbed sleep, and problems with movement (similar to those in Parkinson's disease, which is also associated with Lewy bodies).

Less common again is frontotemporal dementia, in which rogue proteins are again the culprits. There the similarities end, however. Frontotemporal dementia is not closely linked to ageing and has a much stronger genetic component.[8]

So, who gets dementia? The risk factors for Alzheimer's and vascular dementia are not so different from those for stroke. Age is the biggest, with 95 per cent of people with dementia older than sixty-five. Your genes matter a bit, more so for dementias like frontotemporal dementia than others, but generally less than most people think. Black and Asian people are at higher risk of dementia, probably because these populations are more likely to get diabetes and cardiovascular disease, which are themselves risk factors for dementia.[9] High blood pressure, high cholesterol, and being overweight in mid-life are also risk factors – for both vascular dementia and

---

8   For more about frontotemporal dementia and other rare or genetic dementias, see **www.raredementiasupport.org**.

9   The higher average dementia risk among people of Black or South Asian heritage has been assumed to reflect their higher risk of diabetes or high blood pressure. These are in turn caused by the usual mix of genetics and lifestyle, including diet and exercise. But other factors, such as being more likely to live in a poorer area, may also play into the raised dementia risk. Avoidable effects of characteristics such as ethnicity, geography, and disease like this are termed 'health inequalities'. Health inequalities, and how they intersect and overlap, are a really hot topic at the moment.

Alzheimer's – because they too are linked to diabetes and
cardiovascular disease. Appendix 2 covers other risk factors for
dementia that feed into cardiovascular health. It also details
other dementia risk factors that are not linked to cardiovascular
disease.

Avoiding all those cardiovascular risk factors suggests a healthy
lifestyle of physical exercise, diet, no smoking, and not too
much alcohol that reads as a litany of *Thou shalt not*s. On the
upside, a landmark paper published in *The Lancet* in 2020
looked at dementia risk factors along the life course and found
that up to 40 per cent of dementia could be prevented or
delayed. More than a third of dementia is within our own
control.

One of those risk factors for dementia, and one that I didn't
mention above, is low brain resilience, which is sometimes
called low cognitive reserve. This is a relatively new idea, and a
bit different from other risk factors. It's also very closely linked
to puzzles and other ways to stimulate the grey matter. Let's
turn to those next.

4. The puzzles: 1

'Which creature has one voice and yet becomes four-footed and two-footed and three-footed?'

Such is the riddle that the Sphinx, part human and part winged lion, famously poses to Oedipus in Greek mythology. He alone solves the puzzle[1] and the Sphinx ends up killing herself.

Puzzles go way back. The Hindu epic the *Mahābhārata* includes a long philosophical section in the form of a dialogue between two characters, posed as a series of riddles, including 'What is faster than the wind?' (The answer is 'the mind', appropriately enough.) The Egyptians captured puzzles on papyrus as early as 1500 BCE. In the ninth century CE, the scholar Alcuin of York wrote down the first 'river-crossing' puzzle, with its lip-licking wolf, fidgety goat, and passive-aggressive cabbage. Alcuin's brainteaser was for Charlemagne, a puzzle addict who just happened to be Holy Roman Emperor.

---

1   Oedipus answered: 'Man – who crawls on all fours as a baby, then walks on two feet as an adult, and then uses a walking stick in old age.' So, Oedipus wrecks the Sphinx. See Chapter 1 for a more modern take on ageing.

Fast forward to the first jigsaw, invented in the 1760s. The first 'word-cross', as it was then called, came in 1913. Sudoku in its modern form is as recent as 1979. This steady procession of dates speaks to a lasting love-affair with puzzles, maintained over the millennia.

Why does this romance remain when in our online world there are so many other things now teasingly tugging at our leisure time? A J Jacobs writes in his book *The Puzzler* of his nightly emotional odyssey through the *New York Times* crossword, the lows of frustration and despair, the cathartic joy at finding the answer. I hope you can get through the puzzles in *Mind Games* without quite such a white-knuckle ride, but there is surely a thrill in getting the answer, having wrestled with a puzzle for a while.

From struggle comes strength. Here's how.

Puzzle principles

People who regularly engage in cognitively stimulating activities – such as doing puzzles – are likely to see two key benefits.

First, they are more likely to enjoy a slower rate of (healthy) cognitive ageing. In other words they remain sharper for longer, have faster processing speed, and enjoy better attention and memory.

Second, if people who regularly engage in mentally stimulating activities do develop dementia, they are more likely to have a delayed start to their symptoms compared with those who do not. In other words, their brains can tolerate a greater level of disease before that begins to affect them.

We'll see later good evidence that playing a musical instrument and learning a second language, both well-studied forms of mental stimulation, cause physical changes in the brain that make it more resilient. We examine what exactly these healthy changes look like at the level of the network, neuron, and synapse.

Puzzling has not been as well studied as music or language. But we can nonetheless be fairly confident in some principles for how mentally stimulating activities need to be done to reap these benefits.

How should you approach the puzzles in *Mind Games* to have maximum impact on your grey matter? I summarise some principles here, and the suggested puzzle routine in Appendix 1 is designed to follow these.

First, do a variety of puzzles in each sitting. This is to activate different cognitive domains, strengthen different regions and networks of the brain, and hence build a broad base. If you just keep doing the same kinds of puzzle in the same way, you should get better at them – but it might get a bit boring. You are much more likely to see benefits in the real world if you introduce variety: either new types of puzzle or new approaches to puzzles you already do. The gym analogy here is cross-training. For puzzles, the benefits flow from cross-*puzzling*.

Second, do puzzles that are new to you or stretch you. When you've got the hang of a new type, try harder ones or try ones of similar difficulty but give yourself less time. (Sorry, but you can't just stick to the ones you find easy.) In other words, keep challenging yourself. The gym analogy here is moving up to heavier weights.

Third, for benefit the puzzles require sustained mental effort and concentration. No pain, no gain – sorry.

Fourth, do the puzzles regularly. There is no firm evidence, but some experts suggest spending as much time on mentally stimulating activity (not all on puzzles) as the UK physical activity guidelines. That's a lot: 150 minutes each week.

Fifth, you can do the puzzles at any age and still benefit. You might have come to them in mid-life because you want to stay sharp, but there is no bad age[2] to do a mentally or socially stimulating activity. The plasticity of your brain changes as we age but it never disappears. It really is never too early nor too late to start exercising the grey matter. Likewise the gym, though do check with the GP before you go hell-for-leather there.

On the subject of the gym, getting and staying fit are about more than physical exercise. It's the same with mental activity and puzzling: if you want to see sustained changes, or reduce your risk of dementia and stroke, you need to build mental activity into a wider healthy lifestyle. I've summarised this for you in Appendix 2.

---

2   There may be no bad age, but there can be a bad time. Do your puzzles or mental stimulation when you're feeling motivated and not stressed, and when you have the time to yourself without distractions.

Finally, I've focused on cognitive skills, but puzzles also benefit our mood and wellbeing. Every time you close in on a conundrum ('Aha!'[3]) or solve a crossword clue, a little hit of dopamine is released in your brain. Dopamine makes us feel good, and helps us learn better and stay motivated.

In a different way, losing yourself in a jigsaw for a time is almost meditative. That's true of any puzzle that makes you really focus and forget both the outside world and inner worries. Getting lost in a puzzle certainly reduces levels of stress. We know that excess or long-term stress is bad for body and mind, so again puzzles could be helping you age well, through your feelings as well as your 'thinkings'.

The puzzles that follow are arranged according to the cognitive domain that they mainly exercise. Most of the puzzles require use of more than one cognitive domain to solve them, so exactly where each brainteaser appears in the book is a bit arbitrary. But one thing that you'll be exercising a lot in all the puzzles is your executive function. Let's look at that first and then come back to problem-solving at the end of this section.

Executive function

Executive function as a domain is special because it's used to control and coordinate other cognitive skills, especially when

---

3   For the avoidance of doubt, I mean a moment of insight, rather than the Norwegian synth-pop band. A good example might be in Alcuin's wolf, goat, and cabbage river-crossing problem, when Charlemagne clocked that he could bring one of those *back* in the boat as well as take them across.

working towards a goal. Executive function is the 'management' part of your brain. It is usually linked most closely to the prefrontal cortex.

Executive function is what allows you to take a problem-solving approach to each puzzle, to plan a strategy and so on. That planning step might well include a question to yourself: 'Have I come across this kind of puzzle before?'

Some of the puzzles rely on a 'Eureka' moment of sudden insight, but more will involve working through a series of steps. Again, this kind of 'sequencing' or moving from one element of a task to another is part of executive function.

Another key part of executive function that you'll deploy across all the puzzles is attention. This is really closely linked to problem-solving, memory, and learning. If you're not giving something your full attention, then you're like one of my kids 'watching' a film while fiddling with their phone. Ask them at the end of the film about a plot twist and they've probably not registered it. Memorising needs attentionising. (And remember, multitasking is a myth.)

Even when you think you are giving a task your full attention, in practice you are focusing only on certain details – if you doubt this then Google the 'invisible gorilla' psychology experiment.[4]

4   Do check it out. If this famous experiment were a joke it would start, 'So, a guy in a gorilla suit walks into a basketball practice session'. The (true) punchline is that, when people were asked to count the number of passes the basketball players make, half of them did not spot the 'simian' wandering across the court.

That lack of focus is worrying because people will at best commit to memory only a fraction of what was really there, and will recall only a fraction of that. Put like this, it's amazing anyone ever remembers anything at all!

You've already seen how attention and working memory, both vital parts of executive function, are among the brain functions that worsen most as we age. So, toning up both, as you will by doing most of the puzzles, can only be to the good.

Puzzles layout

To show you how the puzzles are exercising different parts of your brain, the following section takes each type of puzzle in turn and follows a consistent approach for each type. First is a thumbnail sketch of the psychology of the cognitive domain being exercised, whether that is memory, word skills or whatever. Next, you'll get a flavour of some of what is happening in your brain when you do that type of puzzle. Then comes a reminder of how that domain is affected by normal ageing, which is your extra incentive to do the puzzles. Each of these sections is followed by a straightforward puzzle of that type as an example.

After these background sections, you'll move on to the first set of puzzles proper, Level 1: Warm-up puzzles, which, as the name suggests, are designed to warm up your brain. Each of the suggested sessions here contains a mixture of puzzle types to exercise a range of different cognitive domains.

After the warm-up things get harder, as you move on to Level 2: Step-up puzzles. This is to keep you challenged. If you're

working through the text and puzzles from cover to cover, you
then get a well-earned break from the puzzles to read a bit more
about the brain. After that, you will progress to some pretty
tough puzzles – Level 3: Buckle-up puzzles, again containing a
mix of puzzle types to exercise a range of domains. These are
followed by the hardest puzzles in *Mind Games*. I've called this
section Level 4: Don't-give-up puzzles, as these are really meant
to stretch you.

Memory puzzles

Memory is a many-splendoured thing. It comes in five or so
types, but is usually split first into short-term and long-term
memory. The latter is then split again into explicit memory
(where we are aware of recalling the memory) and implicit
memory (where we aren't aware of recalling it, like riding a
bike – try explaining *how* you do that!). For all the different
types of memory to work, we have to first capture ('encode')
the memory, then store it, and finally retrieve it.

What we most often think of as memory – remembering life
events such as holidays, a first kiss, weddings, births, and
deaths – is just one of those five or so types: episodic memory.
These memories can feel really vivid: you might recall the sight
of the beach, the feeling of sand between your toes, the smell of
wet seaweed, and the sound of seagulls. These explicit, long-
term memories 'with us at the centre of them' include
autobiographical memories, the narrative of ourselves over time.

Alas, the evidence is that we're not very reliable narrators even
of our own lives. Our stories differ from what others who were

also there remember, we merge and distort memories and we change them as we repeatedly recall them. Worst of all, we confidently remember things that never even happened to us.[5]

Formation (encoding) of episodic memories requires a working hippocampus. The famous patient Henry Molaison (known as H M) had his inner temporal lobes, including most of his hippocampi, surgically removed to control his epilepsy. After the operation, H M became unable to form new memories of anything that happened to him. His working memory and attention were unaffected, and his autobiographical memories from early life were intact, if a bit devoid of detail. Intriguingly, Molaison's ability to imagine things in the future was also badly affected.

Evidence like this suggests that the hippocampus is the initial site where episodic memories are stored, but over time the hippocampus uploads the components of an episodic event to the cortex – so-called memory consolidation. This process, in which the hippocampus 'teaches' the cortex, can last months and is thought to happen while we sleep. For those memories selected for long-term storage, the eventual result is a memory trace. The consolidation of memories into a long-term storage trace like this requires genes in the nerve cell body to be switched on to make new proteins that act at the synapse. Over

5   For a poetic and personal account of the reconstructive nature of autobiographical memory, check out *Pieces of Light: The New Science of Memory* by Charles Fernyhough (Profile Books, 2012). For more about how unreliable memory is, read Julia Shaw's *The Memory Illusion: Remembering, Forgetting, and the Science of False Memory* (Random House, 2016).

time the neurons in the trace also undergo anatomical changes –
at the dendritic spines and axon terminals – to fully consolidate
the memory.

A long-term memory is then represented as a network in which
the cortical neurons have strengthened synaptic connections
between each other: all those holiday elements become strongly
bound together, a bit like a mind map. Exposure to one element
of that trace, say the smell of seaweed, may then trigger us to
reconstruct the whole memory by bringing all the elements
together. The brain areas that originally captured the memory
are the same ones activated when we recall it. Visual memories
are stored in the visual cortex, for example.

How much the hippocampus is needed to retrieve *remote*
episodic memories is controversial. In people with Alzheimer's,
memories of events earlier in life – especially around
adolescence and early adulthood – can often be recalled better
than more recent events because their retrieval relies much less
on the person's shrunken hippocampus. The more remote
long-term memories may rely less on the hippocampus for
retrieval, but they may also feel washed-out, lacking the colour
of a vividly recalled autobiographical scene. Such was the case
for H M.

But the kind of memory that you're pushing hardest for the
puzzles is anything but long-term: it's your working memory.
That is *very* short-term. Anything held in working memory that
is not destined for long-term storage decays fast – it's retained
for no more than about thirty seconds. The most obvious way
that we try to keep something in working memory is to rehearse
it, as when you repeat a phone number (silently or not) before

you write it down. Another similar way is to refresh the original stimulus, For example, if you're asked to look at a picture and remember as much about it as you can, refreshing the stimulus simply means looking at it again. In both cases you need to maintain attention on the task: if you get distracted and lose focus, the information is lost.

As well as being short-term, working memory is very restricted in how much it can hold at once. That capacity limit for most people is about four to nine items of information, such as digits in a phone number or words in a list. Any more than that and working memory risks spilling over, unless you've deliberately made links between items. Otherwise, if you try to remember something else then the new item kicks out what's already in working memory.

Studies of H M suggested that working memories are not stored in the hippocampus, and modern researchers agree: working memory seems to rely mainly on the prefrontal cortex for manipulating information and the parietal cortex for short-term storage and retrieval of sensory signals. In both areas there is some lateralisation of working memory, with words handled mainly in the language areas in the left side of the brain, and vision and space in the right.[6] To deliver working memory, the prefrontal and parietal cortices combine with other, deeper, brain regions to form the 'frontoparietal network'. This network illustrates how working memory is spread around the brain.

---

6   Remember that lateralisation of language to the left hemisphere and spatial information to the right is seen in almost all right-handed people and in three-quarters of lefties. But in a very few right-handers and a quarter of left-handers the generalisations here won't apply.

What happens to the neurons in this network when you use your working memory is not known for sure. A signal is clearly maintained in the frontoparietal network for a few seconds after the initial external stimulus (or its rehearsal) has gone. But that signal decays quickly and does not rely on new proteins being made. In being so short-lived and not reliant on new proteins, working memory is different from long-term memory.

How memory changes with age varies between the different types. We saw in Chapter 3 that some forms of memory are spared or even get better with the years, such as procedural memories (how to ride a bike or tie shoelaces) and semantic memories (general knowledge). But we also saw that others take a hit as we age: episodic memory a bit (as the hippocampus shrinks) and working memory a lot (as the vulnerable prefrontal cortex shrinks).

As you do the memory puzzles, your working memory will be in overdrive, but you will also be drawing on your semantic memory and probably other types of memory as well. Have a go at this example to get you started.

Sample memory puzzle: Memory facts

Spend a minute or two memorising this list of chemical elements along with their chemical symbols and atomic numbers. Once you think you have memorised the list, turn the page and follow the instructions there.

Gold	Au	79
Zirconium	Zr	40
Potassium	K	19
Sodium	Na	11
Tin	Sn	50
Iron	Fe	26
Antimony	Sb	51
Lead	Pb	82

Can you fill in the gaps below with the missing information that you have just memorised? The list is given in the same order as originally presented.

	Au	79
Zirconium	Zr	_____
Potassium	_____	19
_____	Na	11
Tin	Sn	_____
Iron	_____	26
_____	Sb	51
Lead	Pb	_____

When you go on to do the puzzles, the memory puzzles are dead easy to spot: they have names like 'Memory facts' (as above), 'Memory pictures', and 'Memory list'.

Picture puzzles

Puzzles of this type will give your visuospatial (or 'visual–spatial') skills a workout. *Visual–spatial?* That sounds *compli–cated.* Such skills are vital for getting by in the world. As suggested by the name, visuospatial skills cover two things: how we see and then recognise objects (including other people) and how we relate to and manipulate objects – either in reality or in our mind – in space.

In more concrete terms, visuospatial skills are what we use every day when we recognise a friend's face, when we reach out to pick up a cup or catch a ball, when we do up the buttons on our coat or when we successfully park the car. Without them you'd be lost, literally.

What are the underlying processes behind all that in the brain? Vision is the best understood of all the senses. More than half the cerebral cortex is devoted to it. Light is focused on the retina in each of your eyes and that sends electrical signals down the optic nerves. There is an important stopover at the thalamus, which is a kind of relay station in the brain for sensory information, but the upshot is that the nerve impulses arrive at the back of the brain in the visual cortex of the occipital lobe.

The visual cortex is divided into different regions that start to process different features of whatever it is you're looking at (for example edges, lines, and colour), where that object is in space, and whether it's moving or not. This matters because signals from the visual cortex are soon headed off in different pathways for further processing. Signals about the features of the object are sent down to the back of the temporal lobe, where the ability to recognise and name objects (and, separately, faces) mostly lives. The object is identified by being matched to a semantic (factual) long-term memory. In contrast, signals about space and movement that will result in actions – such as catching a ball – are sent on a different pathway, up to the parietal lobe and the motor cortex for the catch.

If you could watch this happening in an intact brain, you would see signals flowing from each eye across the skull to the occipital lobe, and then from there along two separate pathways back across the brain, either up to the parietal lobe or down to the temporal lobe. From each of those lobes, the signals go on to enter the frontal cortex, which is how they end up in your working memory.

Psychologists argue that working memory includes a 'visuospatial sketchpad', where visuospatial information is held for a few seconds while we manipulate it. When you mentally rotate an image for a puzzle of this type, it's this sketchpad that you'll be using. It relies heavily on the parietal and occipital lobes. Of course, the term 'sketchpad' is only a metaphor: if it were a real sketchpad, who in the brain would be looking at it and where would the signals from *their* eyes be processed?

What is amazing is that your brain can break down and analyse all that information coming in from the eyes and then build it back up to give your conscious self a single, unitary picture. We see a grizzly bear coming towards us at speed, not a mish-mash of brown shapes and hair that keeps getting bigger and bigger. More than that, we hear and maybe smell the bear too, as our brain pulls apart, analyses, and then brings together all the sensory information.

Our senses do this by what you might call educated guesswork. Human brains above all are *prediction machines*. Our senses are not simply giving us their best impression of what the world is 'really' like. Instead, they give us information that we subconsciously interpret based on our own internal models, beliefs, and experience of dealing with the world.

As the bear example illustrates, humans who've passed on their genes are those who have been best able to identify the threat and react in time. Waiting until you have certainty – 'Oh yes, that's *definitely* a bear. I can see its sharp tee—' – may leave your DNA in the grizzly's stomach rather than passed on the next generation.

Surprisingly, most of what we 'see' comes not from our eyes but from our brain filling in gaps. (It's the same for all our senses.) The common saying has it the wrong way round: 'believing is seeing' would be more accurate. This is why magicians trick us so easily.[7] We see what we expect to see and are easily distracted. Optical illusions work for the same reason. Figures 3 and 4 show how easy it is to trick the brain.

---

7   For the mysteries of magic and the psychology that magicians exploit, conjure yourself up a copy of Gustav Kuhn's *Experiencing the Impossible: The Science of Magic* (MIT Press, 2019).

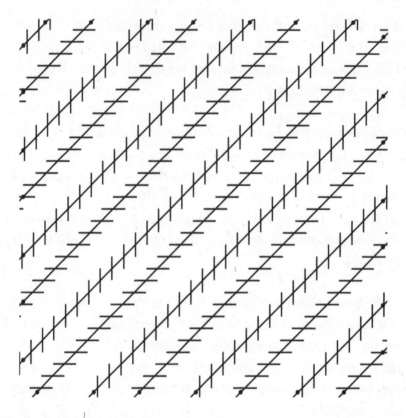

Figure 3: An optical illusion

The diagonal lines running from bottom left to top right are actually
all *parallel* to each other. The brain is misled into not seeing them like
that by the shorter crossing lines. They trick us into seeing the image
more in three dimensions, a bit like a selection of TV aerials coming
out of the page.

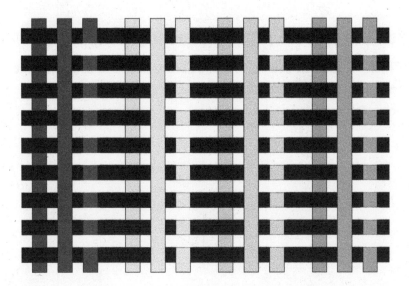

Figure 4: A different optical illusion
The vertical lines within each of the four sets of three are actually all the *same* shade. (If you don't see this effect very clearly, put the book down and view it from a bit further away.) The brain here is misled by 'interference' from the neighbouring black and white horizontal lines, which trick it into seeing shades as lighter or darker.

What happens to our visuospatial skills as we age? The core pathways I've outlined get a bit worse and, as already discussed, our working memory (which includes the visuospatial sketchpad) begins to worsen from as early as age thirty. Our visuospatial skills are also affected by changes in the eyes with age, which means the quality of the data coming into the visual system right at the start begins to deteriorate. So, there's plenty of encouragement, were any needed, to get cracking on some puzzles. Here's an example to have a go at. The answers to all the puzzles are in the Solutions section, starting on p. 287.

Sample picture puzzle: Building blocks

Which of the four sets of blocks could be used to assemble the structure shown at the top of the image? There should be no pieces left over.

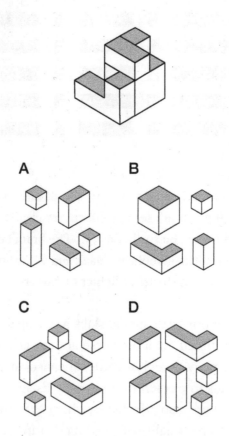

There are lots of picture puzzles in the main puzzle sessions. Look out for more 'Building blocks', but also 'Cube counting', 'Fold and punch', 'Top-down view', and 'Tracing paper' (among others).

Word puzzles

Anagrams, crosswords, wordsearches, word ladders.[8] Puzzles to
give your verbal skills a workout are among the oldest and most
popular. Whether it's Scrabble or Wordle, there's always an
appetite for new ones.

Spoken language comes so naturally that it can be easy to forget
how special it is. People emerge into the world unable to say a
single word but with the capacity to speak any language, so long
as we are exposed to the right environment at the right time.
That this is possible at all comes down to the amazing plasticity
of the infant brain. Learning to read takes more effort, but that's
probably because writing is only a few thousand years old.

The story of how we understand language in the adult brain
goes back to at least the 1860s and 1870s and the work of Paul
Broca and Carl Wernicke. Their lesion studies (see Chapter 2)
revealed how the production of speech relies on one region
(usually) in the left hemisphere (Broca's area), whereas
comprehension of language relies on another in the same

---

8   A word ladder is where you turn one word into another by changing a
letter at a time, always forming a real word at each step. (A
melodramatic example: HATE→HAVE→HOVE→LOVE.) The
invention of word ladders is credited to the prolific puzzler and
Oxford don Rev Charles Lutwidge Dodgson (better known by his
pen name, Lewis Carroll) in 1877. There are several word ladders for
you to descend in *Mind Games*.

hemisphere (Wernicke's area). These brain areas are well
connected, but damage to one does not affect the other. So,
people like Broca's famous patient Louis Leborgne could
understand speech but articulate nothing more than 'Tan, tan'
(hence Leborgne's nickname, 'Tan'). Broca's and Wernicke's are
still viewed as important areas, with wider roles than originally
thought, but it is now known that language relies on a network
that criss-crosses almost the entire brain.

So, what happens in your brain when you do a word-based
puzzle, such as looking for a nine-letter anagram of 'carthorse'?
We saw earlier how the visual pathway starts: when the eyes
scan the page to find the shapes C-A-R-T-H-O-R-S-E, a signal is
sent to the visual cortex for initial processing. What happens
next?

On the underside of the brain, where the occipital lobe meets
the back of the left temporal lobe, is an area that recognises the
letters in that order as a specific word. Its technical name is the
'visual word form area' but it's informally known as the brain's
'letterbox'. The processing here has to cope with a lot of
variation – 'BEAR', 'bear', and even 'bear' written in my terrible
handwriting all trigger our grizzly friend. Unlike the brain
systems for spoken language, the letterbox is thought to have
recently (in evolutionary terms) come into its role, because
writing is such a modern invention compared with vision and
speech.

Signals from the letterbox fire off in several directions, but a key
one is forwards along the left temporal lobe to assign meaning
to the word. Other signals are sent to the lower left parietal lobe

and Broca's area, where comprehension is added in. The connections between the letterbox and language areas get stronger as children learn to read.

We don't know for sure how semantic memory stores words and ideas but they exist in a relational map to each other. So, we store 'bear', knowing that it is 'furry', 'eats meat' and (when we've learned the fact) is a 'mammal', in a 'semantic network'.

And that is only a crude outline of how we read a word that doesn't touch on sentence structure or grammar, which you'll use to understand the puzzle instructions, or humour or irony. You can see why reading exercises so much of the grey matter, and why reading and writing for pleasure are among the cognitively stimulating leisure activities that build brain resilience.

Once you're into the meat of a verbal puzzle you are using your executive function for strategies, your attention to stay on task, and your working memory for manipulating the words or letters. Just like our visuospatial skills had their own compartment in working memory, it's thought that there is a separate place for verbal working memory, which would involve language areas such as Broca's and Wernicke's together with the parietal lobe.

We've seen how semantic memory is one of the brain functions that tends to get better, not worse, with age, as we accumulate knowledge and a wider vocabulary. However, if asked to name as many animals as possible starting with 'B', someone aged seventy may perform less well than a younger person, not because their vocabulary is worse but because of their slower processing speed or worse verbal working memory.[9] Those are the kinds of skills the verbal puzzles will get you working out. The following quick one is to get you started.

---

9   This type of fluid intelligence getting worse with age might not be the
     only cause here. Recent research suggests that the semantic networks
     of older people, where concepts are stored, may be less well
     connected but – intriguingly – more quirky.

Sample word puzzle: Add a word

What one word can be added before all of these to create four new English words?

- MAIL
- STRIP
- SPACE
- LINE

The word puzzles in the main sessions include 'Add a word' (as above), 'Changed sets', 'Connected clues', and 'Word ladder'. You'll also come across some more familiar types such as anagrams, crosswords, word circles, and wordsearches.

Number puzzles

If you're tempted to skip these puzzles because you think you
don't 'do' numbers, please stick with them. They are working
out a lot more of the brain than basic maths does and you can't
avoid numbers anyway – they are *everywhere*.

Everywhere? One neuroscientist counted how many numbers
he saw or heard in an hour on a normal non-working day. Take
a guess.[10]

The story in the brain of how we recognise written numbers is
similar to that for written words. So we look at '1' or '4' on the
page and signals from the eyes start to get processed in the
visual cortex. From there the visual pathway is split, and
recognition of the number '1' requires the semantic memory on
the underside of the rear temporal lobe. In the same way that
recognising a face or a word each relies on a separate area of the
cortex in this region, it's thought that we have a 'number form
area' – like the letterbox, but for numbers.

Like writing, numerals are a recent human invention, but more
so – Arabic numbers (1, 2, 3, etc) are no more than about 1,200
years old. So, the number form area can't have been in the

---

10 The answer, across newspapers, listening to the radio, shopping
     (price tags, car number plates), and so on, was 1,000 numbers an
     hour. See Brian Butterworth's *Can Fish Count? What Animals Reveal
     About Our Uniquely Mathematical Mind* (Quercus, 2022).

evolving human brain for ages, whereas the face recognition area presumably was. We must each learn as young children how '1' means a single item, '2' a pair, and so on. As with words, by learning we commit these number concepts to our long-term memory.

But we don't just see, hear, and say numbers – we *process* them like crazy too. We calculate discounts when we shop, we work out how much food to buy for dinner, we figure out how much time we have to get to the supermarket before it shuts.

As children we learn to distinguish between a big and small number of items well before we are taught formal numbers and the dreaded arithmetic. Psychologists distinguish between 'number tasks', which involve looking at a number or quantity (say, of Smarties) but no arithmetic, and 'calculation tasks', which involve processes such as addition or multiplication. The 'guess the sweets in the jar' game at the village fête is a number task, whereas working out which coins you need to pay for the right to have a guess is a calculation task.

When you are doing a number task, you're exercising two regions of your grey matter in particular. One is in a groove called the intraparietal sulcus that runs along the side of your parietal cortex. The other region is part of the lower prefrontal cortex.

Doing arithmetic calculations draws on additional regions, in particular a much wider area of the prefrontal cortex (including areas linked to working memory). Connections between the number form area and the 'calculation' parts of the parietal cortex get stronger as children develop their maths skills, similar to when they learn to read.

Now while the left–right brain split for language and spatial processing has been known for a while, we've only more recently discovered that how we handle numbers is also lateralised. Simpler number tasks seem to rely more on the right hemisphere whereas more complex calculations rely more on the left. Those leftie calculations may be linked to how we count on our fingers. We usually do this starting (1 to 5) with our dominant hand (right in most people), which is controlled by the opposite side of the brain.

How number skills change with age is not well studied. These puzzles rely on working memory and often semantic memory (general knowledge), which go in different directions as we get older. Beyond that, it may be that our ability to do both number tasks and maths gets better (if slower) as we age. Ability to do number tasks may be preserved because it's more primitive in evolution: small children and quite a few animals[11] can distinguish between five dots and fifteen, but are not able to work out 5 + 15. It's innate rather than taught, and hence harder for ageing to dislodge. Maths skills, as with vocabulary, probably benefit from life experience.

So, number puzzles are helping you in a number of ways, keeping your working memory working and adding to those maths skills you've been honing since your school days. We can't avoid numbers so we might as well learn to love at least *sum* of them! Number puzzle number 1 is next.

---

11 The list of species here is long and includes a lot of primates (gorillas, rhesus and squirrel monkeys, lemurs) as well as dolphins, elephants, birds, salamanders, and fish.

Sample number puzzle: Age puzzle

Amy, Ben, and Claire are siblings of all different ages. Can you
work out, from the clues below, how old each of them is?

- **Claire is not the youngest sibling**

- **In four years, Ben will be twice as old as Amy is now**

- **Claire is three-quarters of Ben's current age**

- **The oldest sibling is thirty-two years old**

As well as more 'Age puzzles', the main puzzle chapters include
other number puzzles. There is a clue in their names, so look
out for 'Number chains', 'Number darts', 'Number pyramid',
and 'Number teaser'.

Logic and reasoning puzzles

Of all the things we do, thinking about a problem in a rational way – as you will especially need to do for the logic and reasoning puzzles – is surely one of the most human. As Aristotle argued, reason is what separates humans from 'brute animals'.

The irony is that, unless you've done a lot of logic puzzles or have Vulcan ancestry, most of us find this kind of brain work really hard. Likewise, in real life we are notoriously sloppy in how we use logic. We make simple errors or take shortcuts that lead us astray. Let puzzle practice make us all more perfect!

One of the most common logical errors that we all make is the 'non sequitur', from the Latin for 'It does not follow'. An example of a non sequitur would be 'Cats have four legs. Rover has four legs. Therefore, Rover is a cat.'

Another everyday logical error, also with a Latin name, is the post-hoc ('after the event') fallacy, which is the mistaken assumption that because event B follows event A, B must have been *caused by* A. An example here would be: 'You kissed a lucky charm before kick-off and your team won. The charm worked!' This gets to the heart of the distinction between correlation (when two things vary in sync) and causation (when one thing really does cause another).

Some of these mistakes in reasoning that we all make come down to a lack of critical rigour, but biases of various types can also trip us up – not least because they often exert their effects without our realising.

So, how do we crack puzzles of logic or reasoning? To solve puzzles of this type, and to some extent of the other types too, you are systematically following a certain set of steps in your brain. First you need to recognise what kind of puzzle it is – or, if it's a new kind of puzzle to you, you're going to need some creativity or insight: an 'Aha!' moment. If you get this first step right, then – with practice – puzzles of the same type can become much easier. (If you don't, expect to spend time barking up some wrong trees.)

Assuming you're not off barking, the second step is planning how you will tackle the puzzle: the sequence of steps you'll follow to find the answer. The final step is working through or executing those steps, which for a logical puzzle will mean applying some set of rules. The specifics of these rules (logical, mathematical, etc) will depend on the puzzle. Get any of these steps wrong and, when you check the solution, you won't get that dopamine hit that comes with a correct answer.

Looked at like this, it's no wonder that logic and reasoning puzzles are going to work out a lot of your grey matter. But which parts?

Psychologists who study creativity distinguish between the 'big C' Creativity of a Manet or Mozart and the more mundane 'small c' creativity of everyday life. The latter covers things such as DIY workarounds, making puns, solving puzzles, and thinking outside the box.

Seeing areas of the frontal lobe light up on scans when people
do creative tasks is not a surprise – creative thinking still needs
to be controlled and directed to be successful. But the
hippocampi are also active. That's because innovative thought
requires us to *imagine* future possibilities, and imagination uses
the same brain regions to look forwards as we use to look
backwards. Back to the past or *Back to the Future* – to the brain
they are more alike than you might think.

If those planning and executing 'goal-directed' steps led you to
think executive function is central to logical problem-solving,
you'd be right. Two parts of the prefrontal cortex (on the upper
outer surfaces and also deeper, on the inner walls of the two
hemispheres) and also the back of the parietal cortex are the
main areas involved. These 'frontoparietal' areas in turn link up
with a host of other brain regions, including different parts of
the frontal lobe as well as much deeper structures. These all
light up on brain scans when people solve a wide range of
problems, so they are thought to represent a general problem-
solving network. This problem-solving network has a lot in
common with the working-memory network outlined
previously.

Although this problem-solving network is deployed in a kind of
general supervisory role across a range of puzzles, it also co-
opts other brain areas and networks to deal with the specifics of
each. You've come across these already, so you know that a logic
or reasoning puzzle based on words will fire up Broca's and
Wernicke's areas in the language network in a way that a logic
puzzle based on numbers won't. The number-based puzzles will
get your number form area and intraparietal sulcus buzzing but
not your language areas. So, solving these puzzles is giving your

problem-solving network a tune-up every time while also working out specific brain areas based on the details of each puzzle.

Attention is also particularly important in this section. Lose focus, make a slip on one of those rules-based logical steps, and you're puzzle toast.

You've seen how even healthy ageing is associated with impaired executive function and attention, which affects the networks for reasoning, mental flexibility, and problem-solving. The prefrontal lobe and the white matter that connects it to the rest of the brain are particularly vulnerable.

This means that if you can keep focused on these puzzles, and stick with the logic without letting other thoughts creep in, you will be giving your logical and reasoning brain a solid workout. And remember, somewhere in your long-term memory may be the solution to a similar kind of puzzle just waiting to be unearthed in an 'Aha!' moment. See if you can dig one out now.

Sample logic and reasoning puzzle: Brainteaser

Three men – Mr White, Mr Green, and Mr Grey – all worked in the same building. They each wore a tie to work every day and, on one particular day, the three men were each wearing a different colour of tie: one wore white, one green, and the other grey.

Mr Green remarked that none of the three men was wearing a tie of a colour that matched their name.

Mr White looked in his briefcase and pulled out a white tie, which he kept in case of emergency. He replaced the grey tie he was wearing with the white one, and then remarked that he was now matching one of the other men's ties, as well as his own name.

Which person was he now matching, and what colour ties had they each had on to start with?

There are a lot of logic and reasoning puzzles in *Mind Games*, including more 'Brainteasers' as well as 'Complete the series', 'Crack the code', and 'Deductions'. The Japanese puzzles Sudoku, Calcudoku, and Futoshiki also rely very heavily on a logical approach.

Level 1: Warm-up puzzles

These first sets of puzzles are the most straightforward in the book. They're designed to gently energise you and to get your brain working in puzzle mode. As you work through the book, things get progressively more complicated.

In case it helps, here are a few general tips that apply to most of the puzzles to help you as you work through them. First, choose a quiet time when you can relax without interruption. (Put your mobile on silent in another room.) Try not to take notes as you work through the puzzles, other than on the logic or reasoning ones.

If you get stuck, take a break or let your mind wander and then try again with a different approach: maybe the numbers are in Roman numerals, maybe 'flower' means a river rather than a rose. Sometimes, as in a maze, you have to go backwards to go forwards again.

For a more complex puzzle, see if you can break it down into smaller parts and work on those. If you focus on an individual part, you might see a principle or pattern that you've missed amid the bigger picture. Finally, if you find you can't do a puzzle, look up the answer in the Solutions section at the back of the book and use that to see how it was done for the next puzzle of that type.

Above all, enjoy!

Session 1

Memory list

Take a minute or so to study this shopping list. When you think you have memorised the list, turn the page and follow the instructions there.

Apples

Bananas

Chocolate chips

Detergent

Eggs

Flour

Grapefruit juice

Haddock

Ice cream

Jam

Can you recall the full list of items in the shopping list by filling in the spaces below? The first letter of each item is given for you, but the list is not in the same order as it was on the previous page.

C_____

I_____

G_____

D_____

J_____

A_____

F_____

B_____

E_____

H_____

Cube counting

How many cubes have been used to build the structure shown?
You should assume that all 'hidden' cubes are present, and that
it started off as a perfect 4×4×4 arrangement of cubes before
any cubes were removed. There are no floating cubes.

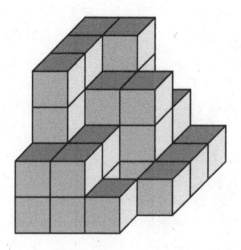

Anagrams

Rearrange each of the following sets of letters to reveal a word you might associate with a yoga class.

1 AMT

2 EOPS

3 CFOSU

4 AAANS

5 EOPRSTU

6 AABCELN

7 ABEGHINRT

8 ADEIIMNOTT

Number chains

Start with the number at the top of each chain, then apply each step of the calculation in turn until you reach the 'RESULT' box. Try to complete the entire chain without using a calculator or making any written notes.

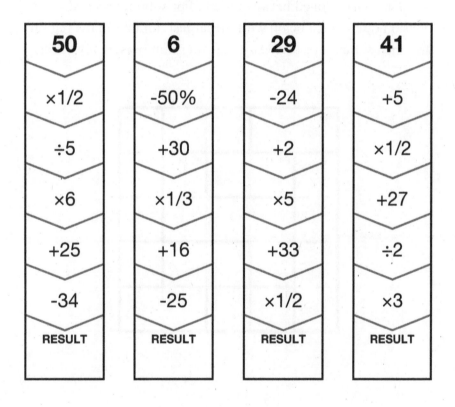

50	6	29	41
×1/2	-50%	-24	+5
÷5	+30	+2	×1/2
×6	×1/3	×5	+27
+25	+16	+33	÷2
-34	-25	×1/2	×3
RESULT	RESULT	RESULT	RESULT

Calcudoku

Place the numbers 1 to 5 once each in every row and column of the grid, while obeying the region totals – regions are outlined in bold. The value in the top-left corner of each region must result when all the numbers in that region have the given operation – addition (+), subtraction (–), multiplication (×), or division (÷) – applied between them. For subtraction and division operations, begin with the largest number in the region and then subtract or divide by the other numbers in any order.

4÷		7+		2–
2÷	6+		900×	
				4÷
8+		1–		
	3×		2÷	

Session 2

Memory pictures

Try to memorise the following images, then turn the page once you're ready.

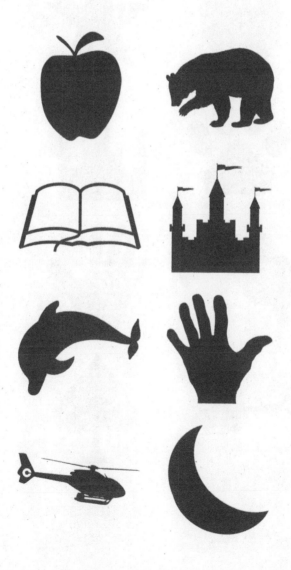

Some of the images have changed. Can you circle all the new images?

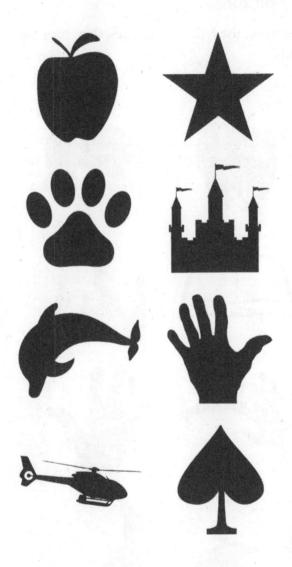

Fold and punch

Imagine folding a piece of paper as shown, and then punching shapes as in the top row. Which of the four options would result were you to then unfold that piece of paper?

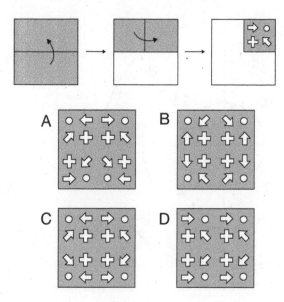

Changed sets

Can you change one letter in each word to create a set of related items? For example, you could change 'HAY', 'COLT' and 'CLOVES' into 'HAT', 'COAT' and 'GLOVES', thus creating a set of cold-weather clothes.

- MANGO

- LIME

- KILN

- BRAVE

- GOLD

Number darts

Form each of the totals below by choosing one number from each ring of the dartboard such that the three numbers sum to the given total.

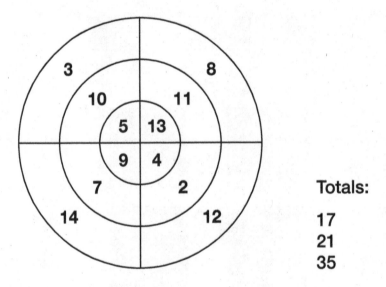

Totals:

17
21
35

Complete the series

Which one of the options below should be placed in the empty square to complete the sequence at the top of the image?

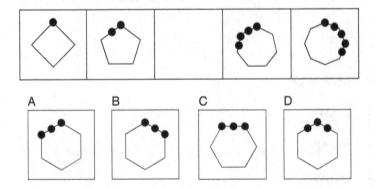

Session 3

Hidden image

Which of the four options conceals the image shown on the left of the puzzle? It may be rotated and rescaled but all elements of it must be visible.

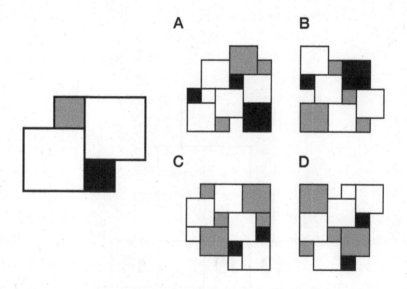

Connected clues

What do the solutions to these clues all have in common?

- City in Florida (7)
- Rubber hockey disc (4)
- Small village (6)
- Female occultists (7)
- Nadir; lowest point (6)

Number pyramid

Complete the number pyramid below by writing a number in each empty brick, so that every brick contains a value equal to the sum of the two bricks immediately beneath it. To the right is a completed pyramid as an example.

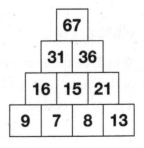

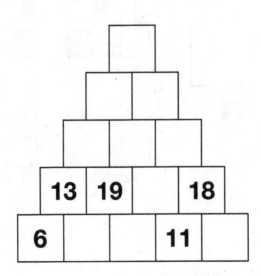

Crack the code

Crack the code used to describe each image, then pick which option should replace the question mark.

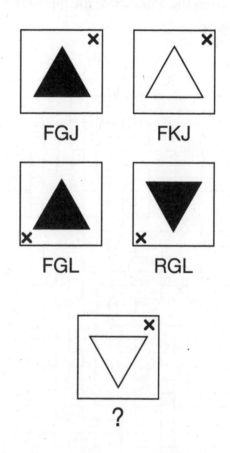

a. RGJ   b. FKL   c. FGR   d. RKJ

Session 4

Maze

Find your way from the entrance at the top all the way to the exit at the bottom.

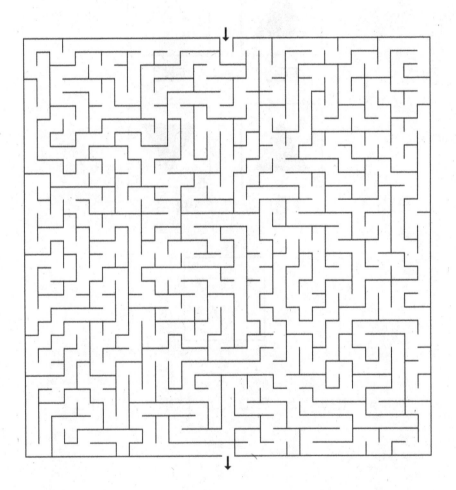

Crossword

Write the solution to each clue in the appropriate boxes (one letter per square).

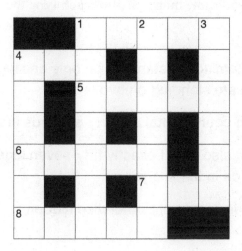

Across
1 Coral island (5)
4 Convulsive muscle twitch (3)
5 Provide food and drink (5)
6 Japanese cuisine (5)
7 Signal 'yes' (3)
8 Histories (5)

Down
1 Blames (7)
2 Acquires (7)
3 Skulked (6)
4 Even chance (4-2)

Number teaser

A wildlife photographer has taken a picture of a lake next to
which several birds are standing. There are two types of bird in
the image: swans and flamingos. Can you use the following
clues to work out how many birds of each type there are in the
image?

- Each flamingo is standing on only one leg, and all the
  swans are standing on two legs

- He can count a total of thirty-six birds in the image

- He can also count exactly fifty-seven legs being
  stood on in the image

- No birds or legs are otherwise hidden

Deductions

Three friends are travelling to meet up for a holiday together.
They are each coming from a different country and each using
a different mode of transport. Can you use the clues below to
work out where each person is setting off from, and using which
mode of transport?

- Peter is travelling by train

- Rudy is travelling from Austria

- Quinn is not travelling by bus

- The person coming from Finland is travelling by boat

- The person travelling by bus is not the one setting off
  from Denmark

Session 5

Reflections

Allowing for a change in scale, which of the four options is the perfect mirror image of the picture on the left-hand side (if the dashed line is the 'mirror')?

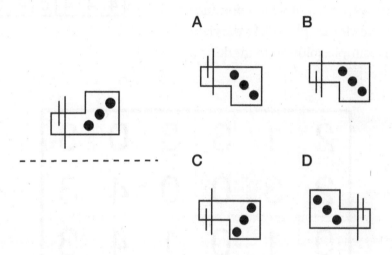

Hidden words

Can you find a hidden colour in each of the following sentences? For example, RED is hidden in 'We <u>are d</u>reamers'.

1   According to legend, the ogre envied the princess so much that he ate her.

2   The woman who broke the window hit every high note in her singing class.

3   I don't use dried basil very much; I prefer to use fresh leaves.

Dominoes

Draw solid lines to divide the grid into a regular set of 0 to 4 dominoes, with exactly one of each domino. A 'o' represents a blank on a traditional domino. Use the check-off chart to help you keep track of which dominoes you've already placed. To the right is an example solution to guide you.

3	2	3	1	0	1
4	1	1	2	0	3
2	0	3	3	3	2
4	1	1	2	0	2
4	4	4	0	4	0

2	1	3	3	0	3
2	3	0	0	4	3
0	1	0	1	4	3
2	1	4	2	4	1
2	1	4	4	2	0

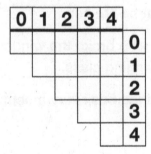

	0	1	2	3	4	
						0
						1
						2
						3
						4

Session 6

Shape count

How many rectangles of all sizes can you count in this image?

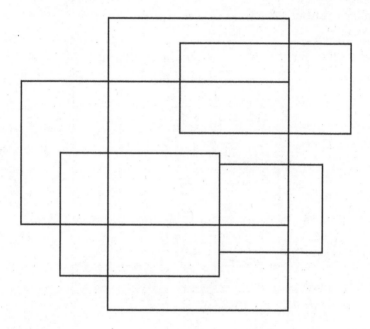

Start and end

What one letter can be added in all the gaps to create four English words?

UTD

_RZ_

VERD

REGAN

Futoshiki

Place the numbers 1 to 5 once each in every row and column while obeying the inequality signs – i.e. the greater than (>) and less than (<) signs. The sign is always pointed towards the smaller number.

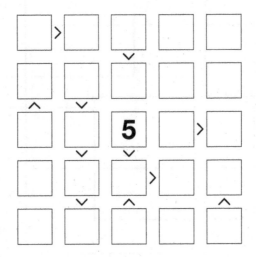

Session 7

Top-down view

Imagine you are viewing the arrangement of blocks shown at the top of the page from above (as indicated by the arrow). Which of the options would be the result?

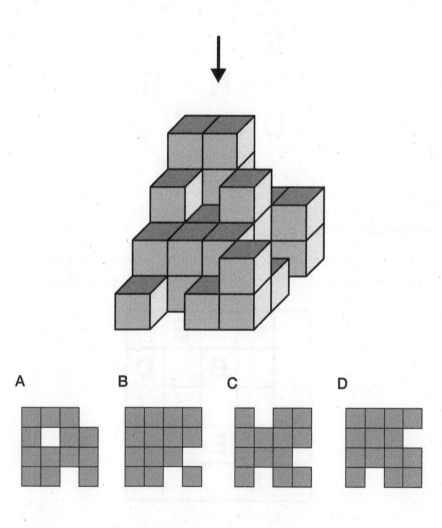

Word circle

How many words can you form that use the centre letter plus two or more of the other letters? No letter may be used more times than it appears in the circle. There is one word that uses all the letters.

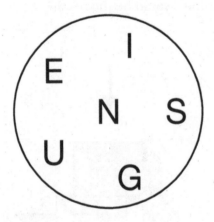

Jigdoku

Place a letter from A to E into each empty square so that no letter repeats in any row, column or bold-lined jigsaw shape.

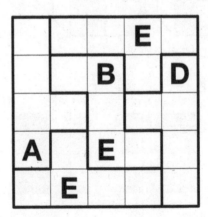

Session 8

Kakuro

Place a number from 1 to 9 into each empty square, such that each continuous horizontal run of white squares adds up to the total given to the left of it and each continuous vertical run sums to the total above it. No number can repeat within any run.

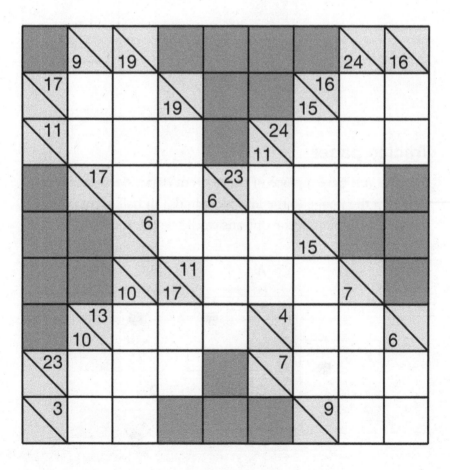

Word ladder

Complete this word ladder by writing a
regular English word at each step. In each
word, you can change only one letter – the
other letters must stay in the same order as
the word above.

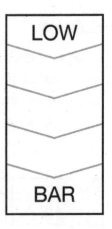

Tracing paper

Imagine you have a piece of transparent paper decorated as
shown in the image to the left. Now fold it in half across the
dotted line. Which of the options would be the result?

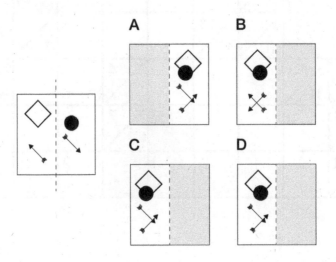

Session 9

Wordsearch

Find the countries written in the grid in any direction, including diagonally. They may also be written backwards.

```
N I N D I A N A M O C
C Y I B Q A T A R F H
E N N A O L Y J N I I
Y I P A H L A N S J N
L N D N S P I R E I A
A E S U A J A V E K S
T B D N O E C Z I M P
I A A R L H I I O A A
N D D T I L O O I A I
S A I L E Q H I R A N
N F E B A Z A M B I A
```

BELIZE	INDIA	KENYA
BENIN	IRAN	OMAN
BOLIVIA	ISRAEL	QATAR
CHILE	ITALY	SPAIN
CHINA	JAPAN	SUDAN
FIJI	JORDAN	ZAMBIA

Shapelink

Draw a series of separate paths, each connecting a pair of
identical shapes. No more than one path can enter any square,
and paths can only travel horizontally or vertically between
squares.

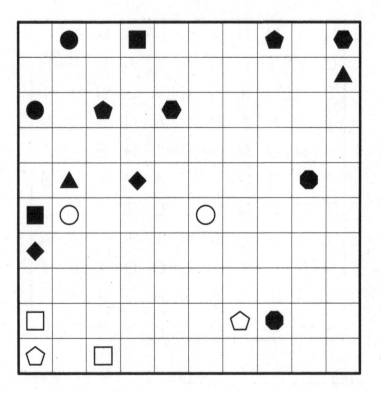

Slitherlink

Connect some of the dots to create a
single loop, so that each digit has the
specified number of adjacent line
segments. Dots can be joined only by
horizontal or vertical lines, and each dot
can be used only once. To the right is a
solved example to guide you.

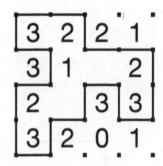

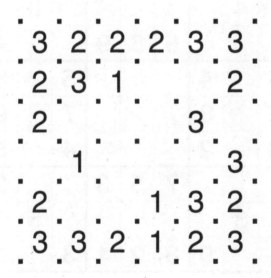

Session 10

Sudoku

Place a number from 1 to 9 into each empty square, so that no digit repeats in any row, column or bold-lined 3×3 box.

		5	1	3	4	6		
	4						8	
7			5	8	9			4
6		4				5		3
5		8				7		9
3		2				4		8
1			7	5	3			2
	3						5	
		9	8	2	1	3		

Touchy

Place a letter from A to F into each empty square in such a way
that no letter repeats in any row or column. Additionally,
identical letters may not be in diagonally touching squares.

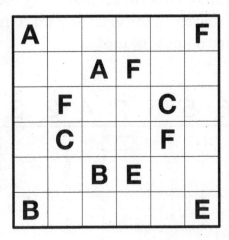

Train tracks

Draw track pieces in some squares to complete a single track
that travels all the way from its entrance in the leftmost column
to its exit in the bottom row. It can't otherwise exit the grid, nor
can it cross itself. Numbers outside the grid reveal the number
of track pieces in each row and column. Every track piece
must either go straight or turn a right-angled corner, and all
given track segments must be used.

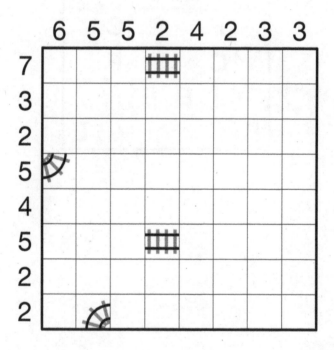

Level 2: Step-up puzzles

The puzzles in this section are harder than the warm-ups, so expect to be doing heavier mental lifting. Again, they're arranged with a mixture of puzzle types in each session. If you complete all the puzzles in each suggested session, you're tuning up most of your grey matter in one sitting. That's a good workout!

Session 11

Memory facts

Spend a couple of minutes studying this list of Olympic athletes, their sports, and the year in which they won a gold medal in that sport. Once you have familiarised yourself with the list, turn the page and follow the instructions there.

Beth Shriever	BMX racing	2021
Duff Gibson	Skeleton	2006
Frida Hansdotter	Skiing	2018
Hamish Carter	Triathlon	2004
James Cracknell	Rowing	2000
Lindsey Jacobellis	Snowboarding	2022
Michael Phelps	Swimming	2008
Nicola Adams	Boxing	2012

Now that you have memorised the medal-winning details, see if you can fill in the blanks below. The list is *not* in the same order that it was originally presented in.

_____	Snowboarding	2022
Beth Shriever	_____	2021
Duff Gibson	Skeleton	____
_____	Swimming	2008
Frida Hansdotter	_____	2018
Hamish Carter	Triathlon	____
_____	Rowing	2000
Nicola Adams	_____	2012

Building blocks

Which of the four sets of blocks could be used to assemble the structure shown to the left of the image? There should be no pieces left over.

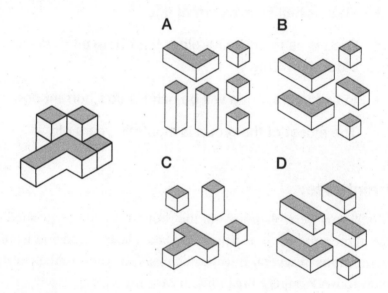

Add a word

What one word can be added before all of these to create four new English words?

- LORD
- FILL
- SLIDE
- LOCKED

Age puzzle

Dom, Eddie, Frida, and Greg are all different ages. Can you work out, from the clues below, how old each of them is?

- Frida is half Dom's current age

- Greg is as many years older than Dom as Eddie is older than Greg

- In two years, Frida will be half Eddie's current age

- The eldest of the group is eighteen years old

Brainteaser

Two friends were planning out the route of a trip they wished to take in the summer. The trip would take place by rail and would feature stops in several European cities. Can you use the clues below to work out the final itinerary for the trip?

- Berlin was not the last stop on the trip

- Lisbon would be visited immediately after Madrid, but neither was the first or last stop on the itinerary

- Prague would be the sixth stop on the trip

- Copenhagen would be visited later than Zurich and Barcelona, but not immediately after either

- Paris would be visited earlier than Barcelona, but not immediately before

- Madrid would be the second stop

- There would be one stop between the stops in Zurich and Berlin

Session 12

Memory list

Take a couple of minutes to study this list of names. When you think you have memorised it, turn the page and the follow the instructions there.

Samira

Margot

Paolo

Sanjeev

Emily

Jonathan

Amani

Helena

Alexander

Jenny

The list of names has been repeated below, although now in alphabetical order. In addition, three names have been replaced with different names. Can you circle the three new names, then write in the missing names?

Alexander

Amalia

Amani

Helena

Jenny

Jonathan

Magdalene

Patrick

Samira

Sanjeev

_____

_____

_____

Cube counting

How many cubes have been used to build the structure shown? You should assume that all 'hidden' cubes are present, and that it started off as a perfect 4×4×4 arrangement of cubes before any cubes were removed. There are no floating cubes.

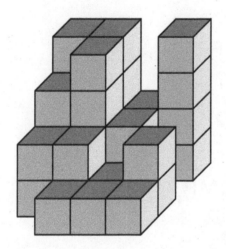

Anagrams

Rearrange each of the following sets of letters to reveal an
animal you might see on a safari.

1 ILNO

2 ABERZ

3 AIKOP

4 AAILMP

5 AGHORTW

6 AEFFGIR

7 AEEHLNPT

8 CEHINOORRS

Number chains

Start with the number at the top of each chain, then apply each step of the calculation in turn until you reach the 'RESULT' box. Try to complete the entire chain without using a calculator or making any written notes.

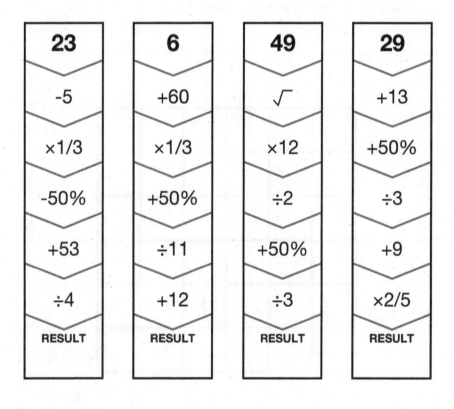

23	6	49	29
−5	+60	√	+13
×1/3	×1/3	×12	+50%
−50%	+50%	÷2	÷3
+53	÷11	+50%	+9
÷4	+12	÷3	×2/5
RESULT	**RESULT**	**RESULT**	**RESULT**

Calcudoku

Place the numbers 1 to 6 once each in every row and column of the grid, while obeying the region totals – regions are outlined in bold. The value in the top-left corner of each region must result when all the numbers in that region have the given operation – addition (+), subtraction (−), multiplication (×), or division (÷) – applied between them. For subtraction and division operations, begin with the largest number in the region and then subtract or divide by the other numbers in any order.

5+		90×	6+	4×	12×
3÷					
10+			20×		3−
	2−		1÷	72×	
6+	9+	6+			
				3×	

Session 13

Memory pictures

Try to memorise the following images, then turn the page once you're ready.

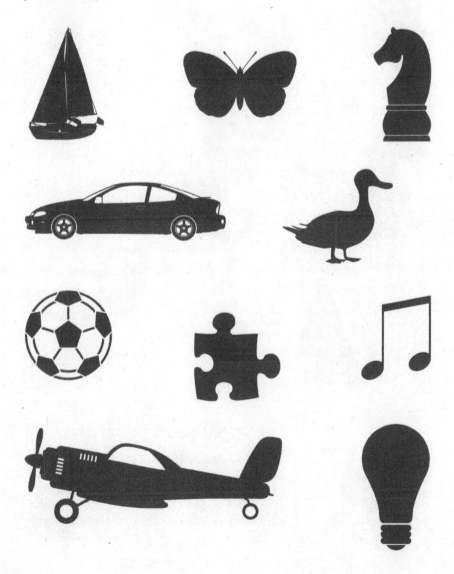

Some new images have been added. Can you circle all the new images?

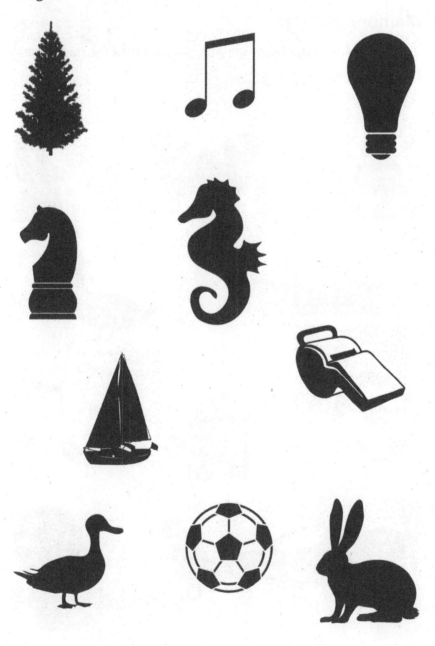

Fold and punch

Imagine folding a piece of paper as shown, and then punching shapes as in the top row. Which of the four options would result were you to then unfold that piece of paper?

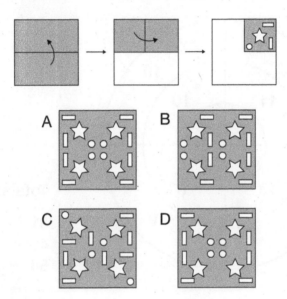

Changed sets

Can you change one letter in each word to create a set of related items?

- NERVE

- JACKET

- COUNT

- DAWN

- DOVE

Number darts

Form each of the totals below by choosing one number from each ring of the dartboard such that the three numbers sum to the given total.

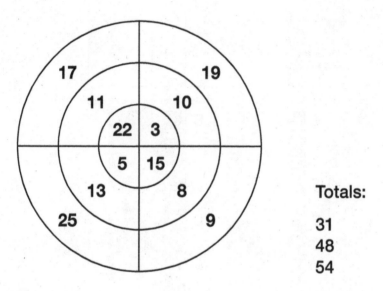

Totals:

31

48

54

Complete the series

Which one of the options below should be placed in the empty square to complete the sequence at the top of the image?

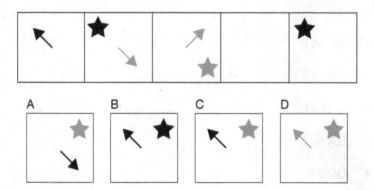

Session 14

Hidden image

Which of the four options conceals the image shown on the left of the puzzle? It may be rotated and rescaled but all elements of it must be visible.

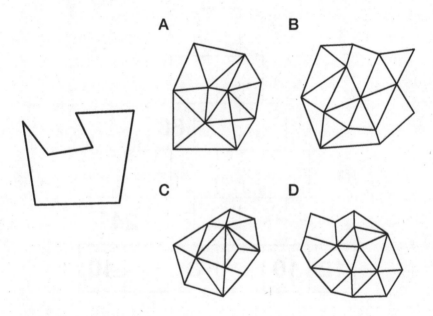

A   B

C   D

Connected clues

What do the solutions to these clues all have in common?

- Light rain (7)

- Steal from one's own company (8)

- Snowstorm (8)

- Blind; amaze (6)

- Noise made by bees (7)

Number pyramid

Complete this number pyramid by writing a number in each empty brick, so that every brick contains a value equal to the sum of the two bricks immediately beneath it.

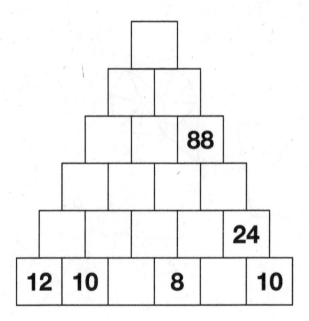

Crack the code

Crack the code used to describe each image, then pick which option should replace the question mark.

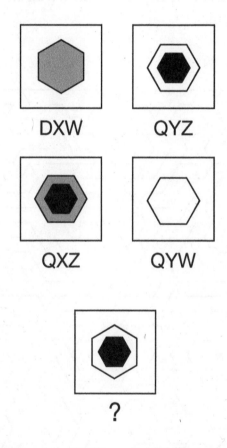

a. QZW   b. DXZ   c. DYZ   d. DXY

Session 15

Maze

Find your way from the entrance at the top all the way to the exit at the bottom.

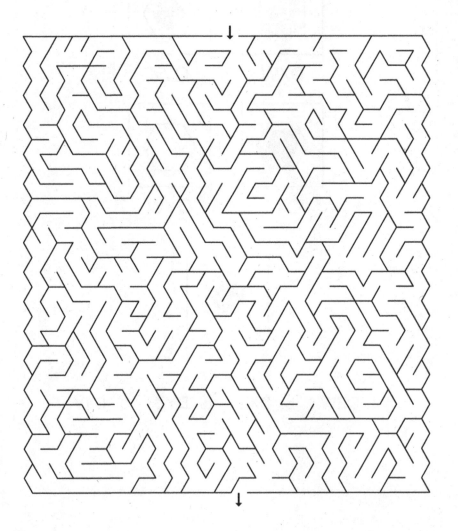

Crossword

Write the solution to each clue in the appropriate boxes (one letter per square).

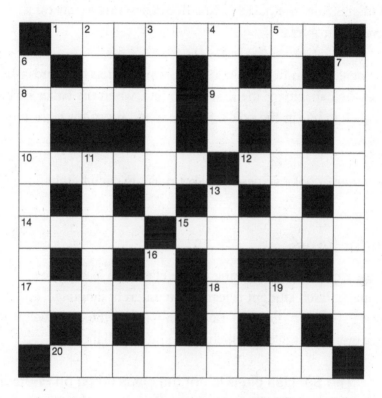

Across
1 Contest opponent (9)
8 More recent (5)
9 Initiate (5)
10 Lots and lots (6)
12 Sharpen (4)
14 Wind up (4)
15 Displacement (6)
17 Punctuation pause (5)
18 Sound (5)
20 Assembly (9)

Down
2 Morning moisture (3)
3 Won (6)
4 Weeps (4)
5 Territories (7)
6 Wrong (9)
7 Purpose (9)
11 Quandary (7)
13 Illicit relationship (6)
16 Clobber (4)
19 Judo level (3)

Number teaser

A baker bakes a batch of cookies every week, always making the same number of cookies. She has a favourite tin that she likes to use to store the cookies, but there are always four that cannot fit, no matter how she packs it. She decides to buy a new tin to solve the problem.

The new tin can fit more cookies, because it has one-and-a-half times the capacity of the first tin. In fact, when the baker's whole weekly batch is in the new tin, there is still room for eight more cookies.

How many cookies does the baker make in each batch?

Deductions

Three students are all taking online classes to learn a new language. Each student is learning a different language, and the classes are all on different days. Can you use the clues below to work out who is taking which class and on what day?

- **The Spanish class is not the class taken on Friday**
- **Chris's class is on Monday**
- **Ali is not the one learning Norwegian**
- **Brian is learning Japanese**
- **One of the classes takes place on Wednesday**

Session 16

Reflections

Allowing for a change in scale, which of the four options is the perfect mirror image of the picture on the left-hand side (if the dashed line is the 'mirror')?

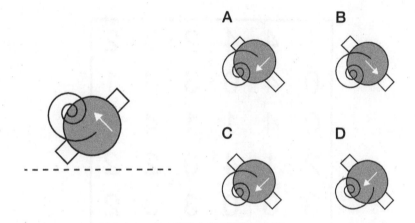

Hidden words

Can you find a hidden country in each of the following sentences?

1   I didn't eat lunch; I left the house too early.

2   Did you spot that cat-like animal? Was it a lynx?

3   I find popping bubble wrap an amazing stressbuster.

Dominoes

Draw solid lines to divide the grid into a regular set of 0 to 4
dominoes, with exactly one of each domino. A 'o' represents a
blank on a traditional domino. Use the check-off chart to help
you keep track of which dominoes you've already placed.

1	4	4	2	3	2
0	4	0	3	3	1
0	4	1	1	4	1
2	1	4	0	2	2
3	0	0	3	3	2

0	1	2	3	4	
					0
					1
					2
					3
					4

Session 17

Shape count

How many rectangles of all sizes can you count in this image?

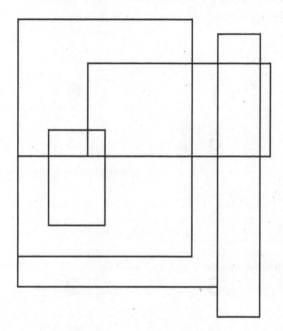

Start and end

What one letter can be added in all the gaps to create four English words?

IVE

AZO

EACTO

ANCOU

Futoshiki

Place the numbers 1 to 6 once each in every row and column while obeying the inequality signs – i.e. the greater than (>) and less than (<) signs. The sign is always pointed towards the smaller number.

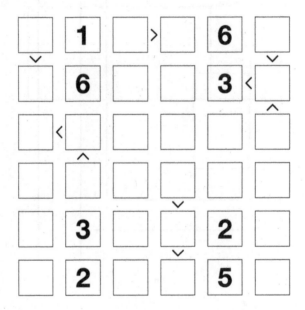

Session 18

Top-down view

Imagine you are viewing the arrangement of blocks shown at the top of the page from above (as indicated by the arrow). Which of the options would be the result?

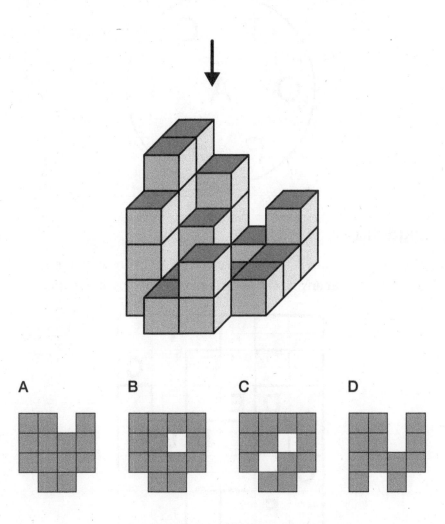

A   B   C   D

Word circle

How many words can you form that use the centre letter plus two or more of the other letters? No letter may be used more times than it appears in the circle. There is one word that uses all the letters.

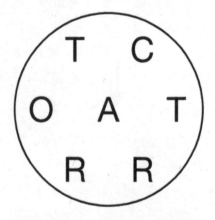

Jigdoku

Place a letter from A to F into each empty square so that no letter repeats in any row, column or bold-lined jigsaw shape.

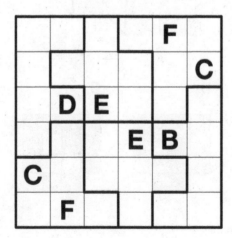

Session 19

Kakuro

Place a number from 1 to 9 into each empty square, such that each continuous horizontal run of white squares adds up to the total given to the left of it and each continuous vertical run sums to the total above it. No number can repeat within any run.

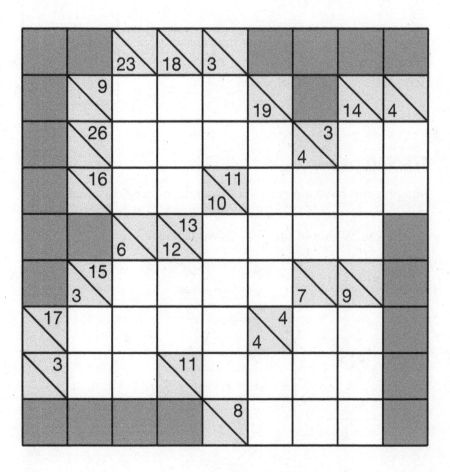

Word ladder

Complete this word ladder by writing a regular English word at each step. In each word, you can change only one letter – the other letters must stay in the same order as the word above.

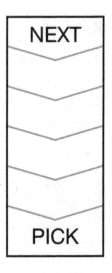

Tracing paper

Imagine you have a piece of transparent paper decorated as shown in the image to the left. Now fold it in half across the dotted line. Which of the options would be the result?

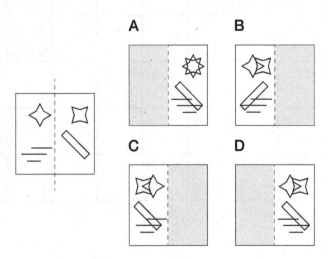

Session 20

Wordsearch

Find the constellations written in the grid in any direction, including diagonally. They may also be written backwards. The middle of the grid is missing, and it is up to you to restore it as you solve.

```
A S I M A S G S U D N I L
S U L V Q P E R S E U S D
V I E I U L M R R O S C C
E R O R A U I P S A A A A
L A V G         P Y R I
A T O O         R B S D
I T O U         I I D P
A I S E         X O A A
R G Q U         D R N O
D A N M R C G P G I R C A
Y S E N E U U O E N A R D
H D U S O S A S G R U S R
A S I S A Y A T D U Y S Y
```

ANDROMEDA	HYDRA	PISCES
AQUARIUS	INDUS	PYXIS
ARIES	LEO	SAGITTARIUS
CAPRICORNUS	LIBRA	TAURUS
CYGNUS	LUPUS	VELA
DRACO	ORION	VIRGO
GEMINI	PERSEUS	

Shapelink

Draw a series of separate paths, each connecting a pair of
identical shapes. No more than one path can enter any square,
and paths can only travel horizontally or vertically between
squares.

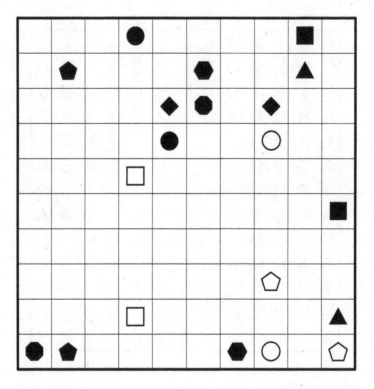

Slitherlink

Connect some of the dots to create a single loop, so that each digit has the specified number of adjacent line segments. Dots can be joined only by horizontal or vertical lines, and each dot can be used only once.

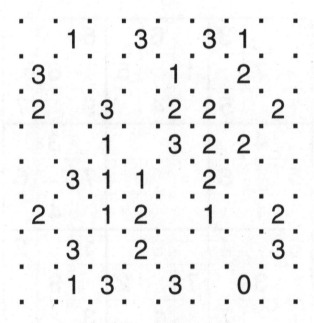

Session 21

Sudoku

Place a number from 1 to 9 into each empty square, so that no digit repeats in any row, column or bold-lined 3×3 box.

		3		6		5		
	7		1		5		6	
1		5		4		9		7
	4						3	
5		8				7		6
	1						4	
6		4		9		1		2
	3		7		2		9	
		7		1		3		

Touchy

Place a letter from A to G into each empty square in such a way that no letter repeats in any row or column. Additionally, identical letters may not be in diagonally touching squares.

A			E			B
		A		D		
	D				A	
B						G
	F				C	
		C		A		
C			B			D

Train tracks

Draw track pieces in some squares to complete a single track
that travels all the way from its entrance in the leftmost column
to its exit in the bottom row. It can't otherwise exit the grid, nor
can it cross itself. Numbers outside the grid reveal the number
of track pieces in each row and column. Every track piece
must either go straight or turn a right-angled corner, and all
given track segments must be used.

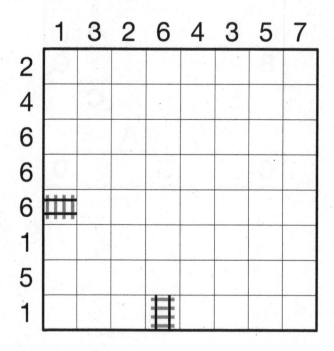

5. The brain strikes back

Adolf Hitler launched Operation Barbarossa, his ill-fated invasion of the Soviet Union, in June 1941, and was from then on fighting to both the east and the west. Your brain is likewise waging war on two fronts.

The first front is a campaign against age-related brain disease, notably stroke and the diseases that cause dementia. The main casualties on this front are neurons. The enemies here are vascular and heart disease, inflammation, and (for dementia) rogue proteins like β-amyloid and tau. With that focus on preventing cardiovascular disease by healthy living, our rallying cry is 'What's good for the heart is good for the head'. This is a vital front for you to fight on, but puzzles are not one of your weapons here. I've summarised the battle tactics in Appendix 2.

The second front is a campaign against not brain disease but the symptoms that disease causes. The casualties here are normal cognition and brain function. The force for good in this battle is a bit harder to grasp. It's the 'resilience' of your brain itself.

This chapter is about this second front against normal cognitive ageing and the symptoms of stroke and – especially – dementia. We will look at these questions:

- What is brain resilience and how does it fight off the symptoms of brain disease?
- How does it develop over our lifetimes?
- How does brain resilience help prevent or delay the emergence of symptoms?
- Which activities are linked to brain resilience?
- How does mental stimulation, such as doing puzzles, contribute to resilience?

Our rallying cry on this second front is 'Use it or lose it'. Some key buzzwords will include 'brain reserve', 'cognitive reserve', and 'neuroplasticity'. As you've seen, puzzles will be part of the weaponry.

But before all that, let's meet some nuns.

Alzheimer's disease without dementia

Nuns might seem an unlikely group in whom to research dementia and its causes, but the Nun Study is among the most famous of its kind anywhere. Researchers in the mid-1980s chose the School Sisters of Notre Dame, Minnesota because the nuns led such similar lifestyles (no smoking, next to no alcohol, similar diet) and all had the same access to healthcare and social support. In other words, they lacked a lot of the messiness that makes research about dementia among a group of women living in the wider world difficult.

In 1986, 678 sisters aged seventy-five or over generously agreed to become guineapigs in the study. Researchers got them to do tests of mental abilities every year and looked closely at their physical health too. Importantly, the nuns agreed to donate their brains for research when they died. That combination of annual assessments over time and autopsy findings, for sisters with and without cognitive decline or dementia, was key.

The poster girl of the Nun Study is one Sister Mary, who was born way back in 1892. She was a lifelong teacher, reader, and social mixer. When Mary died aged 101, she had just scored well on annual cognitive tests, and she remained sharp, alert, and vivacious to the end.

Now some people age better than others, so in itself this was not a big deal. The surprise came in Sister Mary's pathology report: her brain was riddled with plaques and tangles, just like you would see in someone who had died with Alzheimer's disease. Yet Sister Mary had no dementia symptoms. This disconnect between pathology and symptoms – Alzheimer's (brain) disease without dementia – is what research into brain resilience and cognitive reserve seeks to explain.

Now, we saw in Chapter 1 how centenarians may be genetic outliers, and one nun doesn't make a theory. Fortunately for that theory, lots of other studies worldwide have now assessed thousands of people (not just nuns) as they have aged – in some cases getting dementia – and then looked at their donated brains. These studies show that Sister Mary was not a one-off: in a fair few people who live into old age without getting dementia, autopsies show neuropathological changes (Alzheimer's plaques and tangles, Lewy bodies, cerebral infarcts) in their brains.

The number of people like this varies between studies and the degree of brain pathology. Up to about a third of older people have moderate neuropathology but no dementia symptoms. The fraction with severe neuropathology and no symptoms is lower – maybe one in ten – but reflect on that: up to 10 per cent of people with *severe brain pathology* are symptom-free.

This, then, is the battle on that second front: we fight to hold symptoms back by building up brain resilience. Sister Mary had won this battle because her high brain resilience, probably linked to her mentally and socially active lifestyle, kept dementia symptoms at bay. (Had Mary lived to 110, she may have got dementia, but that's not certain.)

What is this near-magical brain resilience? How does it hold back symptoms to delay the onset of dementia even in the face of sometimes severe brain disease? And how can we all get more of it?

Brain resilience

Brain resilience is like gravity: we can see its effects, but we're not sure *how* it works. It was first proposed to explain the disconnect between symptoms or abilities and the amount of brain disease in people like Sister Mary.

There is another side to brain resilience to do with healthy brain ageing. Brain resilience might explain why some people's cognitive functions decline more quickly than those of others as they age, even without disease. Someone with higher brain resilience here would have better cognitive function than an average healthy person of the same age. Their age-related cognitive decline – all those changes to processing speed and attention that we saw earlier in Chapter 3 – has been slowed.

Brain resilience sounds just great – where can I get some? Researching brain resilience involves coming at the topic from lots of different angles: animal studies, brain scans or other measurement of markers of change in humans, and asking volunteers to complete tests of brain function before and after an intervention. But brain resilience is built up over a lifetime, so some of the most informative studies are those in which large groups of people living in the community have been followed for many years.

Some of these so-called longitudinal cohort studies are world famous and have been running longer than most academic careers.[1] Many participants in such studies have submitted to extensive recording of their mental and physical health as well as their lifestyles over time. In some (like the Nun Study), participants have also volunteered to donate their brains when they die to further this research.

Together, longitudinal cohort studies have shown links between brain resilience and a range of lifestyle activities. What you do with your time massively affects how well your functional brain

---

1 The more famous longitudinal dementia cohort studies include the Nun Study and the related Religious Orders Study (both in the USA), and the Honolulu–Asia Aging Study of men of Japanese heritage. The UK has its own Lothian Birth Cohorts, the English Longitudinal Study of Ageing, and the Whitehall studies.

health changes with age. Most studies have focused on resilience, cognitive decline, and the risk of dementia, but there is a lot of interest in brain resilience and stroke too, particularly where stroke affects cognition or language. Resilience and recovery from traumatic brain injury[2] has also been investigated. What do the studies show?

Brain resilience over the lifespan

One of the things that emerges really clearly is that brain resilience is linked to education. Yes, that pesky word 'linked' again. There are many studies showing that an activity is *associated with* higher brain resilience but far fewer studies showing – from 'before' and 'after' measurements – that an activity *increases* brain resilience (or a proxy for it).

The link between brain resilience and education is strongest for formal schooling – school, college, and university – earlier in life. This makes sense, because that's when learning is usually most structured and intensive, and it's also when the brain is at its most responsive to stimulation (see Chapter 7 for why). It may seem a surprise that something you did decades ago can affect your health in later life so much, but it's true: the more years spent in formal education, the more brain resilience you seem to build up and the better your chances of avoiding dementia as you age.

---

2   I'm not going into it in this book, but you may be aware of the growing links found between traumatic brain injury and some forms of dementia, notably 'chronic traumatic encephalopathy'. These links are a particularly active research topic in contact sports such as football, rugby, American football, and ice hockey.

In addition, people who by mid-life have jobs with a lot of complexity, such as crunching data or managing and influencing people, tend to have better brain resilience. In at least one study, working for longer and hence retiring later was linked to a reduced risk of dementia.

Job complexity is linked to formal education because more complex work often requires more qualifications. These are combined into the story of an apocryphal Oxford don. (Why is it *always* Oxford?) Her higher level of education and presumed occupational complexity give her higher brain resilience in later life. So, when she gets Alzheimer's, she gets it at an older age and then symptoms progress more rapidly than expected. This is the 'compression of morbidity' we first came across in Chapter 1. There is no suggestion that the don's greater brain resilience lengthens her overall lifespan, but it does lengthen her *healthspan*.

You might be worrying now that you weren't such a star at school – we all develop at different rates and in different ways – and hence your chance to increase your brain resilience has passed. Fear not! There is plenty of evidence that brain resilience in later life – when age-related cognitive decline becomes more noticeable and when those forces of neuropathological evil are stepping up – reflects both what happened in the first two or three decades of life *and* activities taken up since, in middle and later life. It's never too late to start puzzling!

Importantly, there is evidence that mental activities in mid- and later life are linked to brain resilience in later life, irrespective of your education or occupation. Brain resilience can be affected by doing different things at different times along the lifespan. Your early years matter, but they don't need to hold you back.

The kinds of mid- and later-life activities that are linked to better cognitive ageing and delayed onset or lower risk of dementia are leisure and social activities that are 'cognitively demanding'. In other words, activities that make you think hard and flex the grey matter, or things that encourage lifelong learning. That's a long list. It includes reading, writing for pleasure, playing a musical instrument, learning a second language, playing cards and board games, making art, doing crosswords, and – thankfully, as you're reading this book – solving puzzles.[3]

A paper from 2022 included thirty-eight studies of different activities and enough people (over 2 million) to tease apart the benefits of mental stimulation from social stimulation (see later in the chapter) and physical activity. The combined results showed that doing cognitively stimulating activities in middle to late life reduced a person's risk of dementia by on average nearly a quarter compared with not doing them.

A similar figure emerged from the English Longitudinal Study of Ageing, which is collecting data every two years from 12,000 people older than fifty. Engaging in cognitively stimulating activities reduced dementia risk by 26 per cent compared with not, everything else taken into account. Among people without dementia followed up for fifteen years, time in education and

---

3   Some studies of brain resilience have explored whether watching TV is cognitively stimulating. On balance, and without looking at the types of programmes, the consensus is that it is not.

greater job complexity reduced dementia risk more than doing cognitively stimulating leisure activities did. The overall message from a wide range of studies on mentally engaging activities is clear: use it and you're significantly less likely to lose it.

In separate studies, cognitively demanding leisure activities help with *healthy ageing* as well as dementia risk. Cognition in people doing such activities was better in later life and in the areas hit worst by age-related cognitive decline: memory, processing speed, and executive function.

Whether some activities are better at building brain resilience than others is unclear. So, just keep doing what you enjoy for now. And if you've come across the claims made for computer brain-training games, check out Appendix 3 to see if they really are linked to brain resilience.

In some ways, that lack of evidence as to what works is helpful because it gives you choice. What if the evidence said that writing for pleasure was better than doing crosswords, but that's the opposite of what you enjoy? Knowing what's good for you long-term and putting that into practice in the here and now are far from the same thing – or we'd all be teetotal and never eat chocolate.

Activities to build brain resilience

Let's delve into a few items from that list of cognitively demanding activities to learn a bit more about brain resilience. We'll start with some popular puzzles and then move on to two other activities that have been well researched: playing a musical instrument and speaking two languages.

Mentally stimulating activities

One significant finding on puzzles emerged from a study at Exeter University. Researchers there are following up people aged forty or older online over many years to see how their brain function changes with age according to their lifestyles and health. Among more than 19,000 healthy people aged fifty to ninety-three, how often people did word puzzles – from never to more than daily – was very closely linked to their cognitive performance on tests. Attention, information-processing, reasoning, and both working and episodic memory all improved as puzzles were done more often. And age was no barrier: people over sixty-five showed the same pattern as younger ones.

Those better cognitive skills should translate into better brain resilience, though only a lengthy follow-up, which is planned, would show that. The catch is the familiar millstone around the neck of many such studies, a stone engraved with the text 'Correlation is not causation'. In other words, the fact that improved cognition was *linked to* more puzzle use does not prove that puzzling *caused* the improvements. It might have, but it could be that people who were already more attentive, better at information-processing, and so on were drawn to do puzzles more often. That would be an arrow labelled 'CAUSE' pointing in the opposite direction.

Another puzzle study shows promise in unpacking that link. Researchers followed 488 healthy New Yorkers aged seventy-five to eighty-five and asked – among other things – if they did crosswords regularly. Over the next few years, 101 people in the group got dementia but the first signs of it were seen on average 2.5 years later in the cruciverbalists than in those who were not crossworders. This finding was independent of people's level of education, so it was not the case that brain resilience was down to people having more schooling, which led them to do more crosswords. Consistent with the brain resilience theory, once a crossworder had got dementia their symptoms progressed more rapidly. These findings are as if our Oxford don has migrated from Magdalen to Manhattan. And they suggest something powerful is going on: that the crosswording built up brain resilience against dementia. Is this a case of '*Clues* it or lose it'?

Another hugely popular form of puzzle is the jigsaw, which offers a great brain workout: when you do a jigsaw, you're using visual-spatial skills, mentally rotating the pieces for fit, switching attention between different pieces, and holding a lot in your visual working memory – not to mention the motor skills you use to insert the piece in place or the emotional benefits. A 2018 German study on jigsaws bears all this out. Among 100 healthy people aged over fifty, being a lifetime jigsaw puzzler[4] was linked to better performance on tests that measured broad visuospatial skills.

Let's turn to some other activities linked to building high brain resilience: playing a musical instrument and – separately – speaking two languages. These are not necessarily *better* than other activities, but they've been well studied and will reveal some general principles.

---

4 Apparently, people with a passion for jigsaws are known as 'dissectologists' because in the eighteenth and nineteenth centuries jigsaws were called 'dissected puzzles'. 'Jigsaw' simply refers to the fret saw used to cut the pieces.

It's been known for a while that learning and playing an instrument regularly helps build brain resilience. A 2021 study looked at 5,700 people born around 1940 and whose memory was tested in their sixties and seventies. People were asked whether they had played an instrument at different ages and, if so, how often. As well as suggesting that playing an instrument in adolescence helps to delay dementia, this study showed that starting to play an instrument regularly in adulthood was linked to slower cognitive decline. So maybe here our mantra can be '*Music* or lose it'.

Brain resilience and being fluent in two languages – bilingualism – is a bit of a *patate chaude*[5] because the evidence is not of the highest quality. However, the consensus is that being 'actively' bilingual (i.e. using two languages regularly) over many years is linked to better brain resilience. When bilingual people do get dementia, this may be delayed by as much as four or five years compared with those who speak one language, everything else being equal. Importantly, while the benefits of active bilingualism for brain resilience are greatest when both languages are learned from childhood, adults who become actively bilingual also see clear advantages. In fact, being *proficient* in a second language and using it regularly matters more than the age you learned it.

Socially stimulating activities

Away from cognitive challenges, other kinds of activity that boost brain resilience have a more social focus. Again, if you

---

5   I was expecting 'pomme de terre' to feature in the French for 'hot potato', but apparently 'Non'.

pick these up in mid- or later life, you will still reap the rewards. The long list here includes going to the theatre, enjoying concerts or art events, attending religious activities, socialising with friends and family, volunteering, joining discussion groups, travelling, days out, and dancing. As with mental activities, there is no evidence to suggest that you should choose one over another. Do what you enjoy!

Some of these activities overlap in type. Dancing, for example, includes physical activity, so think of that as a two for one. Other activities in these lists combine mental and social stimulation, so even that distinction is a bit fuzzy. Playing Scrabble with friends or sharing a particularly tricky puzzle with a partner is both mentally challenging and socially stimulating.

Nuns featured at the start of the brain-resilience story, but regular religious practice even without being a 'professional' is another activity that could protect against cognitive decline and dementia. What 'religious practice' means varies enormously in different belief systems, but the benefits of religiosity seem to persist across a wide range of faiths. As I touch on below, being part of a supportive community and the benefits for mental health – less anxiety and depression, better coping with stress – are surely part of the reason. All of these are linked to lower dementia risk. In a similar social vein, living with a partner in mid- to late life seems to reduce your risk of dementia. The flip side is you're at higher risk, especially as a man, if you've never married, or are widowed or divorced.

It might seem obvious that doing puzzles or reading would stimulate the brain, but why are social activities so important? It may be partly that social engagement *is* mental stimulation: as social primates, we've evolved to invest in working out what's going on in someone else's head and planning how to react. (Navigating a social event for me is *always* an exercise in problem-solving – a puzzle that I do not always crack, I am often discreetly informed on the way home.)

Having a supportive social network tends to reduce stress and depression and foster a more positive outlook on life, all of which promote healthy brain ageing. In fact, the larger the social network, the better when it comes to limiting cognitive decline. Do we all need to '*Schmooze* it or lose it'?

Principles to build resilience

Where does all this leave us? If you look at enough studies of brain resilience, you see they're mostly telling us the same general things. We came across these in Chapter 4 but they're worth a recap.

First, activities that seem to promote brain resilience best are those that exercise as much of the brain as possible. Practically, that means that if you want to build up brain resilience you should do a range of different activities. Mix up cognitive, social, and physical stimulation. That's also the reason that the puzzles in this book are designed to exercise different cognitive domains. Variety is the spice of brain life and which specific activities you do may matter less than doing a mix. As Fun Boy Three and Bananarama sang, 'It Ain't What You Do . . .'.

Second, while being stimulated helps, for most benefit you need to keep activities *challenging*. Stretch yourself to do harder things. Easy might be fun, but it's not helping you. Third, the activities should require sustained mental effort or *concentration*. You've got to work at things.

Fourth, you will have to do these activities *regularly* and spend a lot of time on them – you can't learn an instrument or a new language in a few sessions, let alone actually get good at them. So, across all your mental activities, we are talking hours, not minutes, each week. Fifth, if you're going to spend that long on an activity, you will need to stay motivated, so choose activities that you *enjoy* so you want to keep doing them regularly. (How much easier was it to learn stuff at school if the teaching was fun?)

Finally, and possibly most importantly, brain resilience is built (or at times lost) across the *whole lifespan*. Formal education can have a large impact in the first two decades, but mid- and later-life leisure and social activities can then overlay this. The earlier in life you can adopt any brain-healthy habit the better. But – remember those puzzlers, musicians, and bilingual people – it really is never too late to start. As the proverb has it, 'The best time to plant a tree is thirty years ago. The second best time is now.'

Did those principles of building brain resilience sound familiar? If you're a gym-goer you might see how close many of them – regular sessions, variety, reps, progression – would apply just as much to a physical workout plan. So, talk of a 'workout' for the brain is more than marketing blurb.

How brain resilience works

I've spoken about brain resilience as a real thing, but how do researchers reckon it actually works? Current thinking is that brain resilience has at least two different components: brain reserve and cognitive reserve.

Brain reserve is about the brain's *structural* resilience. Large brain reserve here would mean a bigger brain or one with more neurons, more branches on them, and more synapses. These factors depend on someone's genetics and development, but also the environment the person has been exposed to and what activities they've done – as set out above. A person's brain reserve is fixed at a given point in time but varies over their lifetime even in normal health, because of the plasticity of the brain.

In someone with more such brain reserve or 'neurobiological capital', the brain can sustain greater loss – more synapses lost to ageing, more neurons lost to disease or injury – before cognitive function is noticeably impaired. A person with high brain reserve who is affected by brain disease or injury just has more brain tissue to lose.

Cognitive reserve is different. The focus here is on the flow of signals around the brain's nerve networks. In practical terms, higher cognitive reserve shows as increased network activity on a functional MRI scan. But, unlike in brain reserve, you would not expect to see anything different due to cognitive reserve alone in a scan of brain tissue structure.

In someone with higher cognitive reserve the buffer against ageing, disease, and injury is thought to happen in two ways. One is that existing neural networks become stronger because the synapses are more effective. The other is that the brain is able to recruit different networks – neural workarounds a bit like traffic diversions – to compensate for ageing, disease, or injury and so maintain mental function and everyday life. As on a real journey, if you've previously taken a back road, then that route is easier to use again when the motorway gets blocked in future. That is a much more active form of resilience than the passive form seen in brain reserve.

Just like brain reserve, cognitive reserve relies on the plasticity of the brain. And just like its sibling, cognitive reserve is shaped by genetic influences and is built up by lifetime stimulation. More stimulation – including more puzzling – creates more effective and more flexible neural networks. As we'll see when we look in more detail at neuroplasticity, 'neurons that fire together wire together'.

I've described brain reserve and cognitive reserve as separate, but they don't work against each other, and an individual may have high levels of one or both together. But both rely on the ability of the brain to change in different ways over time, especially in response to the external environment. That ability to change is neuroplasticity. It's where we'll complete our journey.

But before any of that, here are some more puzzles.

6. The puzzles: 2

You're now heading towards the deep end of the puzzle pool, where you'll need to work harder and build on what you've learned so far. The puzzles towards the end of this section include some real head-scratchers, but stick with them and the rewards from a correct answer will be all the greater.

Level 3: Buckle-up puzzles

These puzzles are the next-to-most challenging in *Mind Games*. As before, they are grouped to work out different cognitive domains at each session.

Session 22

Memory facts

Spend a few minutes memorising this list of Oscar-winning films, along with the category of their win and the year of their release, then turn the page and follow the instructions there.

Nomadland	Best Picture	2020
Coco	Best Animated Feature	2017
Avatar	Best Art Direction	2009
All About My Mother	Best Foreign Language Film	1999
A Close Shave	Best Animated Short Film	1995
Mrs Doubtfire	Best Makeup	1993
Dead Poets Society	Best Original Screenplay	1989
Women Talking	Best Adapted Screenplay	2022

Can you fill in the gaps below with the missing information you have just memorised? The list is *not* in the same order that it was originally presented in.

_____ _____ **1995**

All About My Mother _____ _____

_____ **Best Art Direction** _____

_____ _____ **2017**

Dead Poets Society _____ _____

_____ **Best Makeup** _____

_____ _____ **2020**

Women Talking _____ _____

Building blocks

Which of the four sets of blocks could be used to assemble the structure shown to the left of the image? There should be no pieces left over.

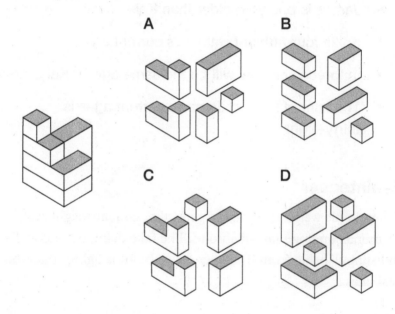

Add a word

What one word can be added before all of these to create four new English words?

- UP
- AXE
- LED
- POCKET

Age puzzle

Hamina, Ivy, James, and Kai are all different ages. Can you use the clues below to work out how old each of them is?

- **James is one year older than Kai**

- **Kai is four-fifths of Hamina's current age**

- **In three years, Ivy will be the same age as Kai is now**

- **The sum of Ivy and James's current ages is thirty-eight**

Brainteaser

A jeweller is weighing a pile of gems that contains eight real diamonds and one fake diamond. The fake diamond is visually indistinguishable from the other gems, but it is lighter than the real ones.

To determine which is the fake, the jeweller plans to use a set of balancing scales to weigh the collection of gems. All the genuine gems are identical, so have exactly the same weight.

In the interests of efficiency, what is the fewest number of times the jeweller must use the scales to guarantee they have identified the fake? Each time they use the scales they place one or more jewels on each side of the balance and then see which way it tilts.

Session 23

Memory list

Spend a few minutes studying this list of animals. When you think you have memorised it, turn the page and follow the instructions there.

Axolotl

Alligator

Anchovy

Albatross

Antelope

Anteater

Aardvark

Ape

Auk

Adder

Arapaima

Ant

Now that you have memorised the list, see if you can write it down in its entirety on the lines below, in the same order that it was originally presented in. If you get stuck, turn back and try to memorise the missing items. Repeat until you have recalled them all.

_____

_____

_____

_____

_____

_____

_____

_____

_____

_____

_____

Cube counting

How many cubes have been used to build the structure shown?
You should assume that all 'hidden' cubes are present, and that
it started off as a perfect 4×4×4 arrangement of cubes before
any cubes were removed. There are no floating cubes.

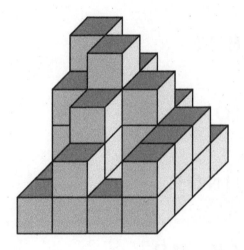

Anagrams

Rearrange each of the following sets of letters to reveal an African capital city.

1 INSTU

2 AABRT

3 ACIOR

4 ABIINOR

5 AAAKLMP

6 AAHIKNSS

7 AHKMORTU

8 ADGHIMOSU

Number chains

Start with the number at the top of each chain, then apply each step of the calculation in turn until you reach the 'RESULT' box. Try to complete the entire chain without using a calculator or making any written notes.

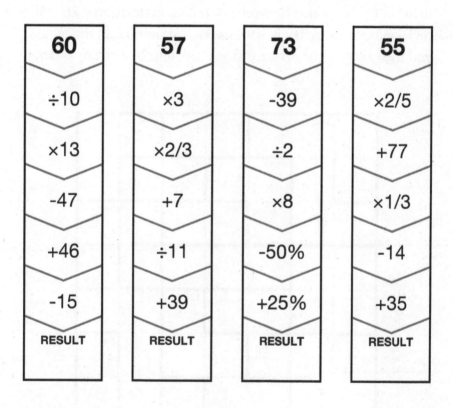

60	57	73	55
÷10	×3	-39	×2/5
×13	×2/3	÷2	+77
-47	+7	×8	×1/3
+46	÷11	-50%	-14
-15	+39	+25%	+35
RESULT	RESULT	RESULT	RESULT

Calcudoku

Place the numbers 1 to 7 once each in every row and column of
the grid, while obeying the region totals – regions are outlined
in bold. The value in the top-left corner of each region must
result when all the numbers in that region have the given
operation – addition (+), subtraction (–), multiplication (×), or
division (÷) – applied between them. For subtraction and
division operations, begin with the largest number in the region
and then subtract or divide by the other numbers in any order.

4–	70×		12×		48×	
		210×		3+		
			24×		12×	8+
1–	5+	1–				
		3–		126×	26+	
1–	6+					6÷
		1–				

Session 24

Memory pictures

Try to memorise the following images, then turn the page once you're ready.

Some of the images have changed. Can you circle all the new images?

Fold and punch

Imagine folding a piece of paper as shown, and then punching shapes as in the top row. Which of the four options would result were you to then unfold that piece of paper?

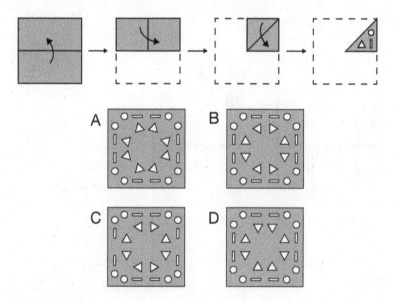

Changed sets

Can you change one letter in each word to create a set of related items?

- RAMEN
- PETROL
- ROSIN
- SCAN
- STARTING

Number darts

Form each of the totals below by choosing one number from each ring of the dartboard such that the three numbers sum to the given total.

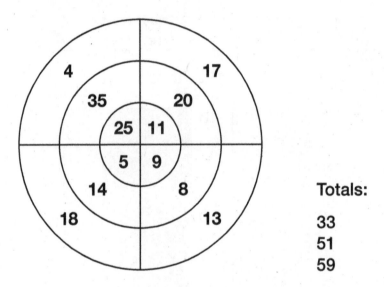

Totals:

33
51
59

Complete the series

Which one of the options below should be placed in the empty square to complete the sequence at the top of the image?

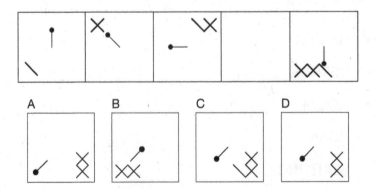

A   B   C   D

Session 25

Hidden image

Which of the four options conceals the image shown on the left of the puzzle? It may be rotated and rescaled but all elements of it must be visible.

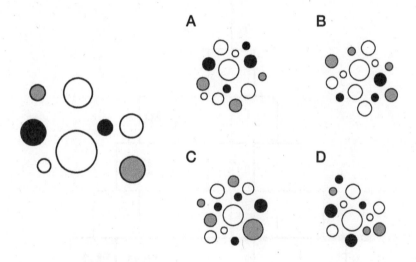

Connected clues

What do the solutions to these clues all have in common?

- Hairstyle with short front and sides but long back (6)

- Place to rest temporarily (5)

- Only; bottom of the foot (4)

- Four-stringed guitar (4)

- Lucky or chance occurrence (5)

Number pyramid

Complete this number pyramid by writing a number in each empty brick, so that every brick contains a value equal to the sum of the two bricks immediately beneath it.

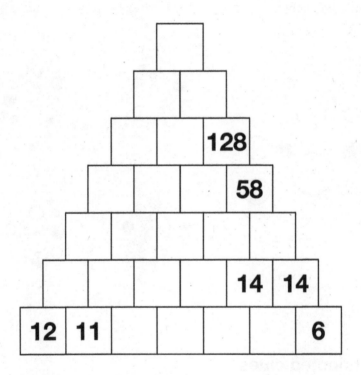

Crack the code

Crack the code used to describe each image, then pick which
option should replace the question mark.

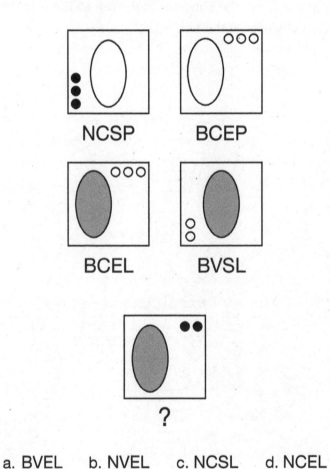

a. BVEL   b. NVEL   c. NCSL   d. NCEL

Session 26

Maze

Find your way from the entrance at the top all the way through the circle to the exit at the bottom.

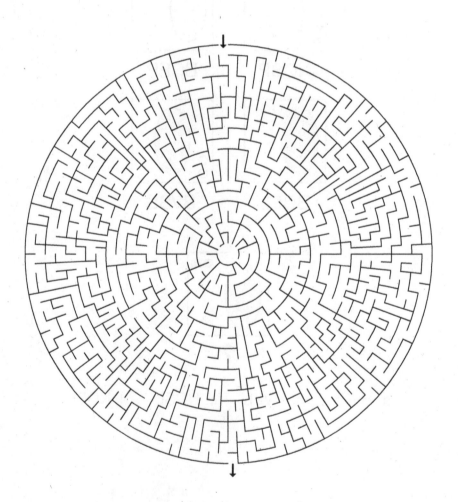

Crossword

Write the solution to each clue in the appropriate boxes (one letter per square).

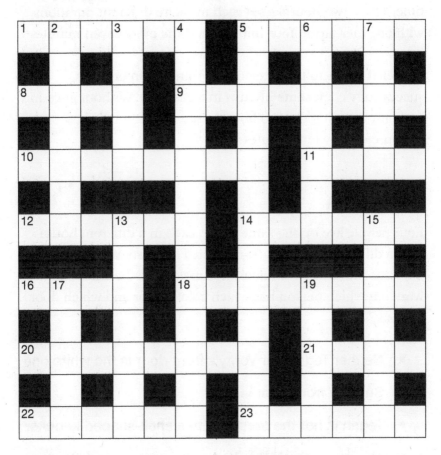

Across
1 Take in (6)
5 Reach a destination (6)
8 Electric light source (4)
9 As one (3,2,3)
10 Erroneous (8)
11 Hope (4)
12 Lobbed (6)
14 Auxiliary track section (6)
16 Make changes (4)
18 Alarms (8)
20 Plant specialist (8)
21 Ninth letter of the Greek alphabet (4)
22 Globe (6)
23 Put right (6)

Down
2 Bestial (7)
3 Circle around (5)
4 As contrasting as can be (5,3,5)
5 Business organizer (13)
6 Rejuvenated (7)
7 Action words (5)
13 Appalling act (7)
15 Made ineffective (7)
17 Sag (5)
19 Expression (5)

Number teaser

A chef has two hourglasses in their kitchen but – due to a power cut – currently has no other way of measuring the passage of time. These two hourglasses each measure different durations, with one measuring four minutes and the other seven minutes.

The chef needs to time exactly ten minutes, in order to successfully cook some biscuits in a gas oven. Without guessing, and only by using the two hourglasses, how can the chef measure exactly ten minutes?

Deductions

Four people live on the same street, each in a different house with a different-coloured front door. They also each have a different shape of door knocker. Can you use the clues below to work out which person has which colour door and which door knocker?

- Neither Tegan nor Verity's front door is the white one

- Sunita's front door is red

- Tegan is not the person with a shell-shaped knocker

- The green front door has a knocker shaped like a claw

- The house with the blue door has a knocker shaped like a fox

- Verity's door is not blue

- Ursula's door knocker is in the shape of a leaf

Session 27

Reflections

Which of the four options is the perfect mirror image of the picture on the left-hand side (if the dashed line is the 'mirror')?

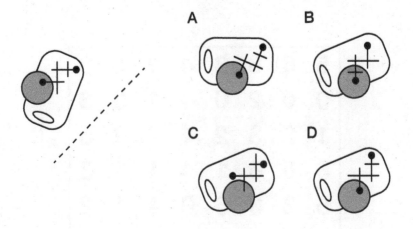

Hidden words

Can you find a hidden fruit in each of the following sentences?

1   There's a phone call I'm expecting before lunch, so I might be hard to reach.

2   Is 'thumb' an anatomical term, or is there a more technical one?

3   I usually cheer for the home team, but they played so badly today.

Dominoes

Draw solid lines to divide the grid into a regular set of 0 to 6 dominoes, with exactly one of each domino. A '0' represents a blank on a traditional domino. Use the check-off chart to help you keep track of which dominoes you've already placed.

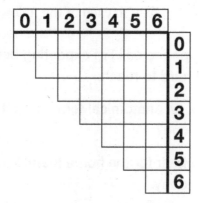

Session 28

Shape count

How many rectangles of all sizes can you count in this image?

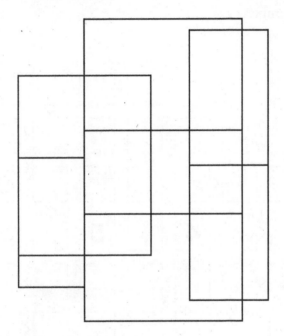

Start and end

What one letter can be added in all the gaps to create four English words?

LIT

RAS

LOP

AGL

Futoshiki

Place the numbers 1 to 7 once each in every row and column while obeying the inequality signs – i.e. the greater than (>) and less than (<) signs. The sign is always pointed towards the smaller number.

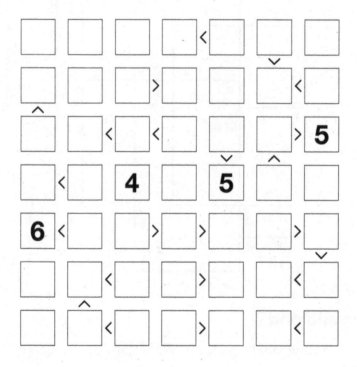

Session 29

Top-down view

Imagine you are viewing the arrangement of blocks shown at the top of the page from above (as indicated by the arrow). Which of the options would be the result?

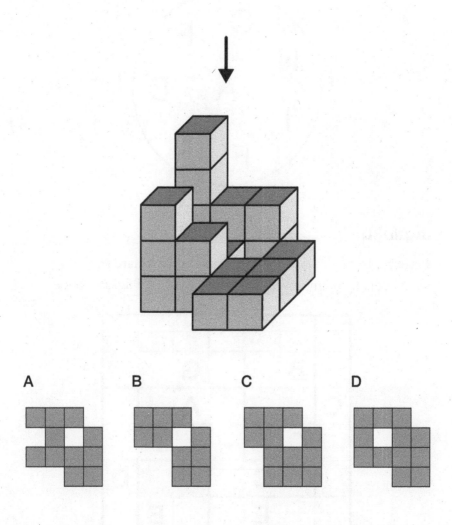

A   B   C   D

Word circle

How many words can you form that use the centre letter plus two or more of the other letters? No letter may be used more times than it appears in the circle. There is one word that uses all the letters.

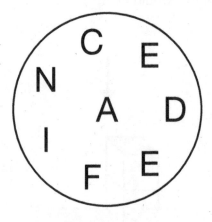

Jigdoku

Place a letter from A to G into each empty square so that no letter repeats in any row, column or bold-lined jigsaw shape.

Session 30

Kakuro

Place a number from 1 to 9 into each empty square, such that each continuous horizontal run of white squares adds up to the total given to the left of it and each continuous vertical run sums to the total above it. No number can repeat within any run.

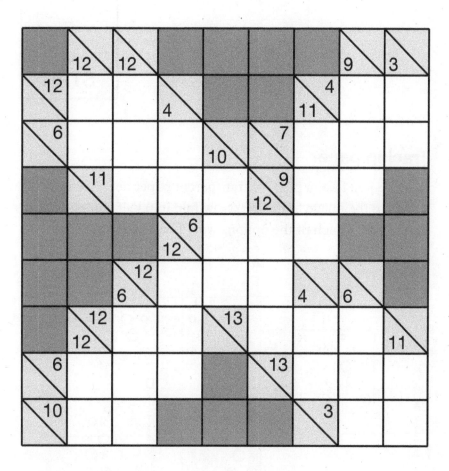

Word ladder

Complete this word ladder by writing a
regular English word at each step. In each
word, you can change only one letter – the
other letters must stay in the same order as
the word above.

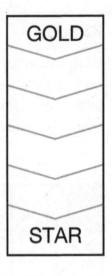

Tracing paper

Imagine you have a piece of transparent paper decorated as
shown in the image to the left. Now fold it in half across the
dotted line. Which of the options would be the result?

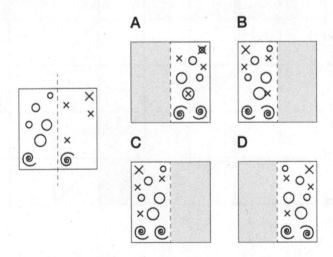

Session 31

Wordsearch

Find the listed birds written in the grid in the stereotypical 'shape' of a bird, as shown by the example word VULTURE. The words may read either from left to right or from right to left.

```
R  L  X  O  I  P  I  W  I  N  G  G  O  L  O
E  A  A  B  E  L  I  L  D  B  A  O  P  P  T
W  A  L  R  A  B  L  P  O  M  N  S  N  A  S
N  O  N  L  I  W  G  N  I  W  M  I  R  C  I
W  T  T  R  R  M  S  N  I  U  F  U  E  R  H
I  S  D  O  U  K  L  P  S  N  L  D  H  E  E
G  P  O  R  I  T  E  U  A  P  S  S  R  L  S
M  R  E  B  O  N  E  N  V  R  T  M  P  O  I
R  R  I  O  P  T  T  R  R  A  O  C  S  S  C
N  N  C  W  S  A  I  P  C  S  S  D  H  R  O
G  P  A  Y  R  N  L  R  W  S  E  A  P  E  C
R  P  O  R  E  O  N  D  E  R  E  S  P  R  R
S  O  A  E  G  I  W  B  C  G  L  O  T  E  S
N  I  R  T  H  A  L  K  A  N  R  O  S  S  S
L  R  S  O  L  A  W  H  N  T  G  R  O  S  E
```

ALBATROSS	OYSTERCATCHER	SPOONBILL
CORMORANT	PASSERINE	STORK
GOLDCREST	ROBIN	SWALLOW
GOOSE	SANDPIPER	VULTURE
HERON	SEEDSNIPE	WAGTAIL
HUMMINGBIRD	SNOWFINCH	WAXBILL
LAPWING	SPARROW	

Shapelink

Draw a series of separate paths, each connecting a pair of
identical shapes. No more than one path can enter any square,
and paths can only travel horizontally or vertically between
squares.

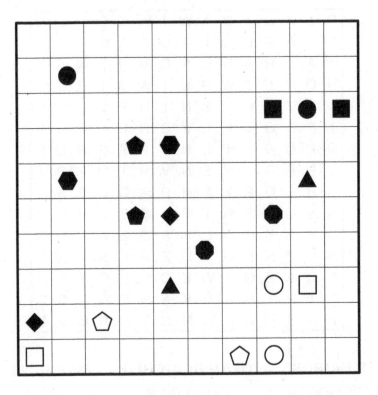

Slitherlink

Connect some of the dots to create a single loop, so that each digit has the specified number of adjacent line segments. Dots can be joined only by horizontal or vertical lines, and each dot can be used only once.

```
  .   .   .   .   .   .   .   .   .   .
    2           1     3     3
  .   .   .   .   .   .   .   .   .   .
    3           1     1     3
  .   .   .   .   .   .   .   .   .   .
  2 2           2           3
  .   .   .   .   .   .   .   .   .   .
    3           3     2
  .   .   .   .   .   .   .   .   .   .
  2 1     2 3     3 1 1
  .   .   .   .   .   .   .   .   .   .
    2 3 0     1 1     0 2
  .   .   .   .   .   .   .   .   .   .
      3     1           1
  .   .   .   .   .   .   .   .   .   .
  3           2           2 3
  .   .   .   .   .   .   .   .   .   .
  1     1     3           2
  .   .   .   .   .   .   .   .   .   .
  2     3     3           2
  .   .   .   .   .   .   .   .   .   .
```

Session 32

Sudoku

Place a number from 1 to 9 into each empty square, so that no digit repeats in any row, column or bold-lined 3×3 box.

3			5		1			9
	9						4	
		7				2		
9			7		4			1
				3				
2			6		8			7
		6				1		
	4						6	
7			8		3			5

Touchy

Place a letter from A to G into each empty square in such a way that no letter repeats in any row or column. Additionally, identical letters may not be in diagonally touching squares.

F						A
		G		F		
	E				G	
	B				A	
		D		E		
A						F

Train tracks

Draw track pieces in some squares to complete a single track that travels all the way from its entrance in the leftmost column to its exit in the bottom row. It can't otherwise exit the grid, nor can it cross itself. Numbers outside the grid reveal the number of track pieces in some rows and columns. Every track piece must either go straight or turn a right-angled corner, and all given track segments must be used.

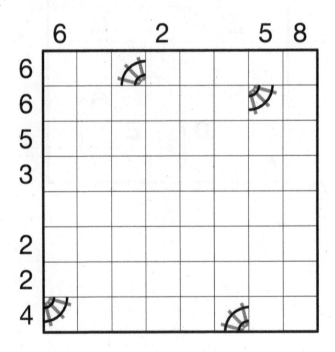

Level 4: Don't-give-up puzzles

The teasers in this section are going to push your puzzling prowess to the limits. That means you'll be getting a really thorough brain workout. Best of luck!

Session 33

Memory facts

Spend a few minutes studying this list of plants and animals and their scientific names. Once you've familiarised yourself with the list, turn the page and follow the instructions there.

Apple tree	*Malus domestica*
Wild cherry	*Prunus avium*
Chicken	*Gallus gallus domesticus*
English oak	*Quercus robur*
Fox	*Vulpes vulpes*
Giraffe	*Giraffa camelopardalis*
Hazel	*Corylus avellana*
Human	*Homo sapiens*
Scots pine	*Pinus sylvestris*
Tiger	*Panthera tigris*
Wolf	*Canis lupus*

Now that you have memorised the list, see how many of the
Latin names you can recall. The list is *not* in the same order that
it was originally presented in.

Fox   _____

Scots pine   _____

Wild cherry   _____

Wolf   _____

Chicken   _____

Human   _____

English oak   _____

Giraffe   _____

Apple tree   _____

Hazel   _____

Tiger   _____

Building blocks

Which of the four sets of blocks could be used to assemble the structure shown to the left of the image? There should be no pieces left over.

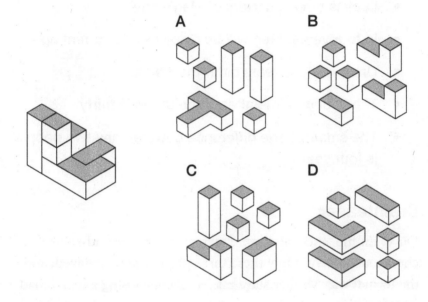

Add a word

What one word can be added before all of these to create four new English words?

- BACK
- POWER
- PLAY
- SHOE

Age puzzle

Lucy, Meg, Nora, and Omar are all different ages. Can you use the clues below to work out what age each of them is?

- Lucy is three-quarters of Meg's age

- In four years, Meg will be twice Nora's current age

- Omar is eight years older than Nora

- The youngest member of the group is thirty

- The smallest age difference between any two people is four years

Brainteaser

Dave, Emma, and Faisal were taking part in a round-robin chess tournament. Only these three players were involved, and the format was 'winner stays on', so anyone losing a match had to wait their turn until the next game. Can you work out who won the fifth game based on the following facts?

- In total nine matches were played

- Dave played in four games, and lost all of them

- Faisal won two consecutive games, but had no other wins

- Emma lost the first game

Session 34

Memory list

Take a few minutes to memorise this list of random words.
Once you think you'll be able to recall the entire list, turn the
page and follow the instructions there.

Lemon

Mouse

Education

Wedding

Yacht

Magnolia

Yoghurt

Icicle

Speedy

West

Rainbow

Travel

Now that you have memorised the list, see if you can write it out in alphabetical order. To help you, the second letter of each word has been given.

   _ d _____

   _ c _____

   _ e _____

   _ a _____

   _ o _____

   _ a _____

   _ p _____

   _ r _____

   _ e _____

   _ e _____

   _ a _____

   _ o _____

Cube counting

How many cubes have been used to build the structure shown? You should assume that all 'hidden' cubes are present, and that it started off as a perfect 4×4×4 arrangement of cubes before any cubes were removed. There are no floating cubes.

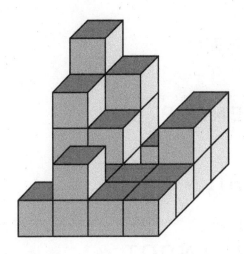

Anagrams

Rearrange each of the following sets of letters to reveal a Renaissance artist.

1 BCHOS

2 AIINTT

3 AAEHLPR

4 BEHILNO

5 ADELLNOOT

6 EINOORTTT

7 BCEIILLOTT

8 ACEEGHILLMNO

Number chains

Start with the number at the top of each chain, then apply each step of the calculation in turn until you reach the 'RESULT' box. Try to complete the entire chain. You can make written notes here if you need to.

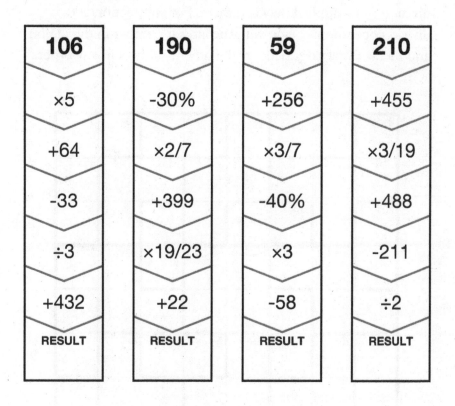

106	**190**	**59**	**210**
×5	-30%	+256	+455
+64	×2/7	×3/7	×3/19
-33	+399	-40%	+488
÷3	×19/23	×3	-211
+432	+22	-58	÷2
RESULT	**RESULT**	**RESULT**	**RESULT**

Calcudoku

Place the numbers 1 to 8 once each in every row and column of the grid, while obeying the region totals – regions are outlined in bold. The value in the top-left corner of each region must result when all the numbers in that region have the given operation – addition (+), subtraction (−), multiplication (×), or division (÷) – applied between them. For subtraction and division operations, begin with the largest number in the region and then subtract or divide by the other numbers in any order.

2−	2÷		6+	3−		13+	
	48×				240×		11+
20×		56×			15×		
	26+		540×			56×	
		2×					6×
1−	25×		19+	2−		8×	
							48×
16×		28×			3÷		

Session 35

Memory pictures

Try to memorise the following signs, then turn the page once you're ready.

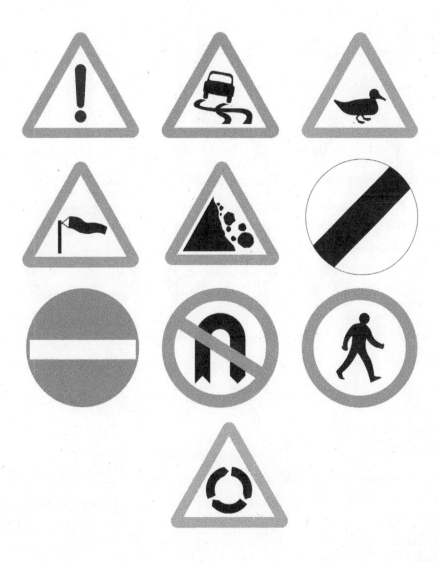

The contents of the signs have been removed. Can you restore them all?

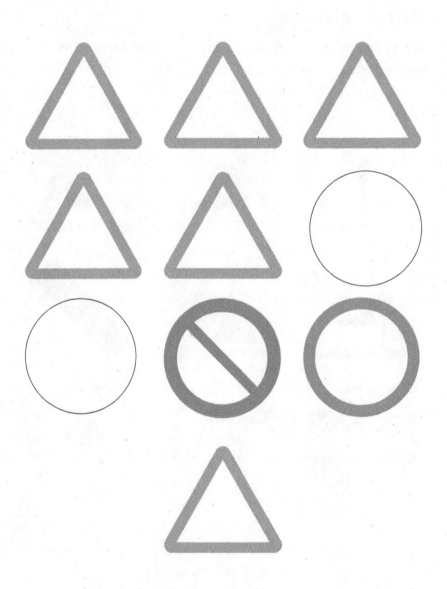

Fold and punch

Imagine folding a piece of paper as shown, and then punching shapes as in the top row. Which of the four options would result were you to then unfold that piece of paper?

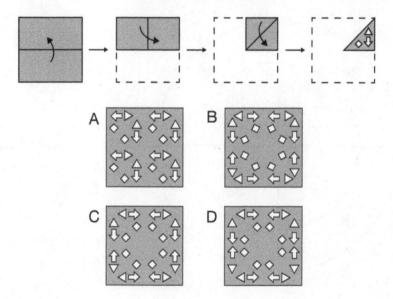

Changed sets

Can you change one letter in each word to create a set of related items?

- PARTS
- PLAGUE
- HOME
- TUNES
- BARN

Number darts

Form each of the totals below by choosing one number from each ring of the dartboard such that the three numbers sum to the given total.

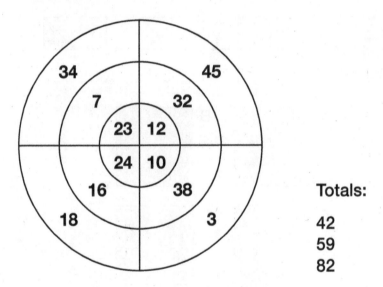

Totals:

42

59

82

Complete the series

Which one of the options below should be placed in the empty square to complete the sequence at the top of the image?

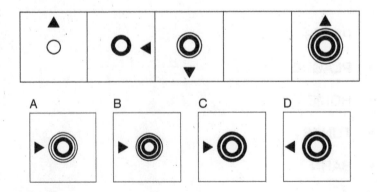

Session 36

Hidden image

Which of the four options conceals the image shown on the left of the puzzle? It may be rotated and rescaled but all elements of it must be visible.

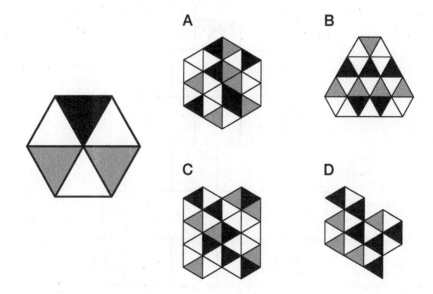

Connected clues

What do the solutions to these clues all have in common?

- Better; higher ranking (8)

- British queen (8)

- Exsanguinated (4)

- Asteroid impact site (6)

- Festive cervid? (8)

Number pyramid

Complete this number pyramid by writing a number in each
empty brick, so that every brick contains a value equal to the
sum of the two bricks immediately beneath it.

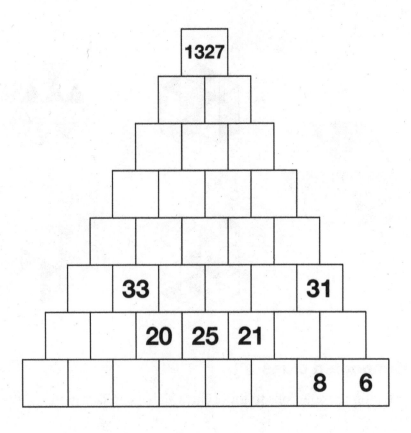

Crack the code

Crack the code used to describe each image, then pick which option should replace the question mark.

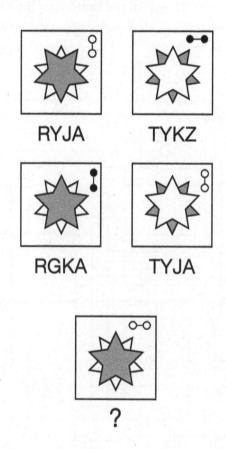

a. RYKZ   b. TYJZ   c. RGJA   d. RGJZ

Session 37

Maze

Find your way from the top to the bottom of the maze. Some paths pass under or over other paths using the given bridges.

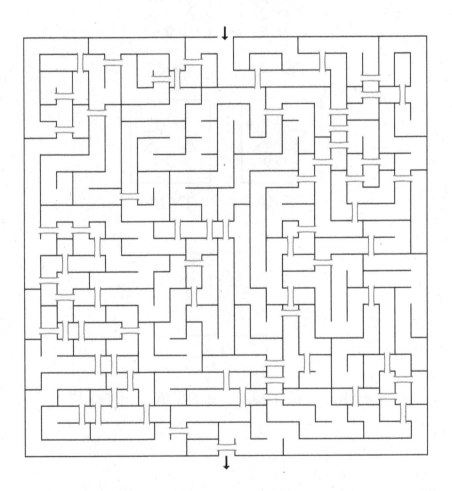

Number teaser

An entomologist has a pet stick insect that seems to have an extraordinary appetite. He placed a large number of green leaves – each of identical size – inside the insect's enclosure, to provide a substantial supply of food.

The entomologist monitored the insect's eating habits very closely. On the first day of monitoring, the insect ate three leaves in total. The next day, it ate five leaves, meaning that the insect ate the same number of leaves as it had eaten the previous day, plus an extra two. This pattern continued, with an extra two leaves on top of the number eaten the day before being consumed on each day.

The first day of monitoring was a Monday, at the start of which 100 leaves had been added to the enclosure. If no additional leaves were later added, how many leaves would the insect have left in the enclosure at the beginning of the following Wednesday, nine days later?

Spiral crossword

Write the solution to each clue into this spiral crossword in the appropriate direction (one letter per box).

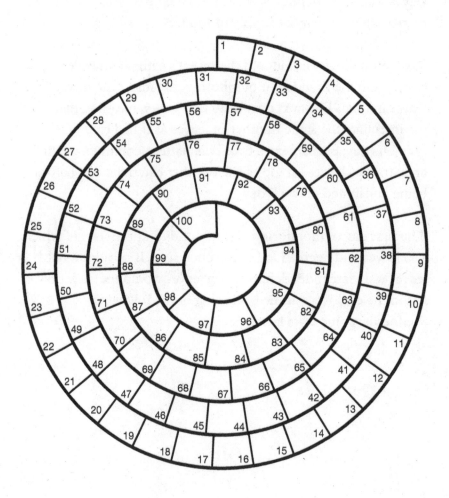

Inwards

1–6	College treasurer
7–11	Poetic lament
12–14	Metal-bearing mineral
15–19	Municipal
20–24	More mature
25–28	'Bother!'
29–31	Like hearts and diamonds
32–36	Lawful
37–41	Truffles, for example
42–44	Doze
45–50	Boxing glove, slangily
51–55	Dominant animal in a pack
56–62	Ocular cleansing lotion
63–67	Sticky ribbons
68–72	Absurd
73–76	Low ground between hills
77–80	Brick oven
81–85	Single things
86–96	Stretchable
97–100	Frozen, with 'over'

Outwards

100–95	Come to a conclusion
94–90	Implied
89–85	Discount events
84–82	Can
81–76	Dissimilar
75–71	Weighed down
70–66	Parsley relative
65–61	Tracks
60–58	Sense of amazement
57–54	'Sure!'
53–48	Pluto used to be one
47–41	Kettledrums
40–38	African antelope
37–34	Masthead pennant
33–29	Senior
28–22	Played the main role
21–18	Mathematical positions
17–11	Sovereign's stand-in
10–8	Hair-styling substance
7–4	Periods of time
3–1	Polish

Deductions

A florist is assembling a bouquet with three different types of flower. Each flower type is a different colour, with all the flowers of that type being the same colour. There are a different number of each type of flower in the bouquet. Can you use the clues below to work out how many of each type of flower is in the bouquet, and what colour each type is?

- There are twice as many tulips in the bouquet as roses

- The number of orange flowers is two-thirds of the number of yellow flowers

- The roses are not the pink flowers

- In total, there are eighteen flowers in the bouquet, including gerberas

Session 38

Reflections

Allowing for a change in scale, which of the four options is the perfect mirror image of the picture on the left-hand side (if the dashed line is the 'mirror')?

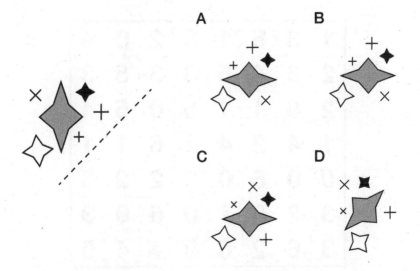

Hidden words

Can you find a hidden animal in each of the following sentences?

1   Some hairdressers give the scalp a careful massage when washing hair.

2   Please don't make the vicar mad, I'll only have to apologise later.

3   Do you have a spare sugar lump, or cup? I need two of everything for a tea party.

Dominoes

Draw solid lines to divide the grid into a regular set of 0 to 6 dominoes, with exactly one of each domino. A '0' represents a blank on a traditional domino. Use the check-off chart to help you keep track of which dominoes you've already placed.

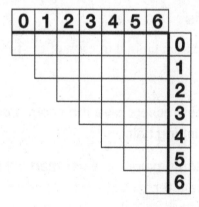

1	3	6	1	5	2	0	4
2	6	4	5	3	3	5	3
2	6	1	1	5	0	5	4
1	4	2	4	4	6	1	1
0	0	6	0	3	2	2	5
3	2	5	1	0	6	0	3
3	6	2	6	0	4	4	5

0	1	2	3	4	5	6	
							0
							1
							2
							3
							4
							5
							6

Session 39

Shape count

How many rectangles of all sizes can you count in this image?

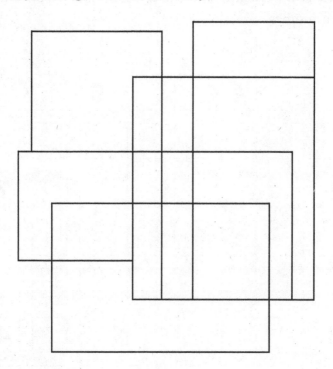

Start and end

What one letter can be added in all the gaps to create four English words?

ITHDRA

ORKFLO

INNO

IDO

Futoshiki

Place the numbers 1 to 8 once each in every row and column
while obeying the inequality signs – i.e. the greater than (>)
and less than (<) signs. The sign is always pointed towards the
smaller number.

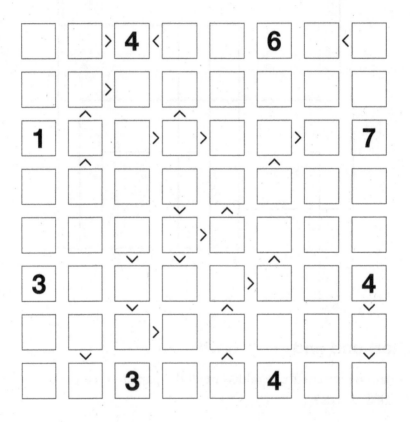

Session 40

Top-down view

Imagine you are viewing the arrangement of blocks shown at
the top of the page from above (as indicated by the arrow).
Which of the options would be the result?

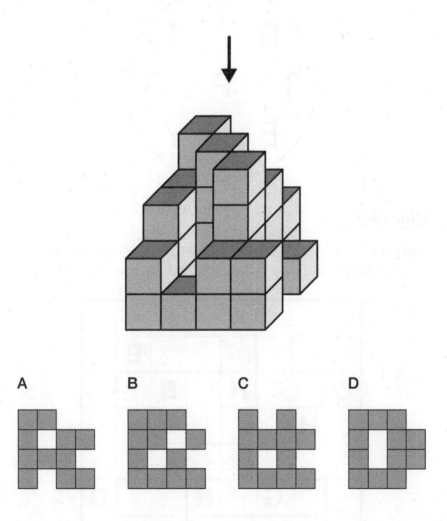

A   B   C   D

Word circle

How many words can you form that use the centre letter plus two or more of the other letters? No letter may be used more times than it appears in the circle. There is one word that uses all the letters.

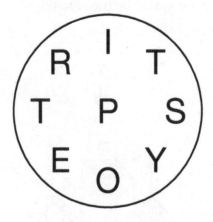

Jigdoku

Place a letter from A to H into each empty square so that no letter repeats in any row, column or bold-lined jigsaw shape.

			A		F		
						B	
C			H		B		
	H						
						F	
		G		H			D
	C						
		H		A			

Session 41

Kakuro

Place a number from 1 to 9 into each empty square, such that each continuous horizontal run of white squares adds up to the total given to the left of it and each continuous vertical run sums to the total above it. No number can repeat within any run.

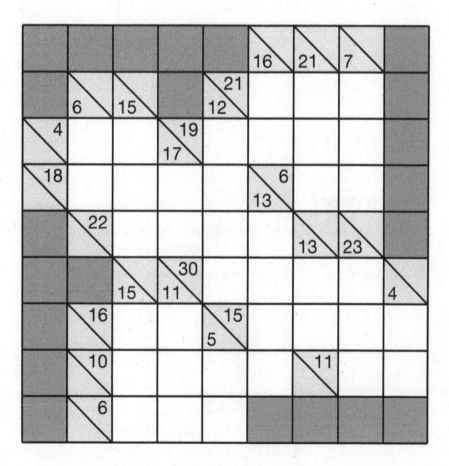

Word ladder

Complete this word ladder by writing a regular English word at each step. In each word, you can change only one letter – the other letters must stay in the same order as the word above.

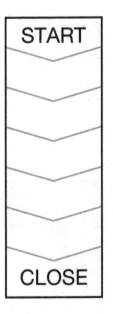

Tracing paper

Imagine you have a piece of transparent paper decorated as shown in the image to the left. Now fold it in half across the dotted line. Which of the options would be the result?

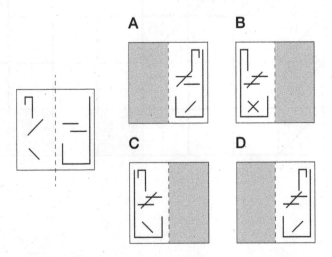

Session 42

Wordsearch

Find the listed shapes written in the grid in spirals, as shown by the example word RECTANGLE. They always read outwards from the centre, but the spiral may be at any of four rotations.

```
L E P E M G U A R E P H O V L
C C G L L E Q S E R S E L A A
R I M A P L E C E X E R N D E
M E U R A O N O H A Y R I C R
A Y M A R G E N O G P A L Y C
N E E N W R A A C D I M A G O
O D E T E N P T A M A P T P N
G A C I K O E H G A N G N E T
T E L B U S T N O T R L R W E
G C T M R O N D E C E E E G D
N O A O H M D A R T E O I D P
N O G E N A I E H R N Z T R L
R E L E S T P S E Z I E P A E
L N G T R A I E P T U D E A A
I I N A I E L L A R M P U E R
```

CIRCLE	HEXAGON	RHOMBUS
CONE	KITE	SPHERE
CYLINDER	OCTAGON	SQUARE
DECAGON	OVAL	STAR
DIAMOND	PARALLELOGRAM	TRAPEZIUM
ELLIPSE	PENTAGON	TRAPEZOID
HEART	PYRAMID	TRIANGLE
HEPTAGON	RECTANGLE	WEDGE

Shapelink

Draw a series of separate paths, each connecting a pair of
identical shapes. No more than one path can enter any square,
and paths can only travel horizontally or vertically between
squares.

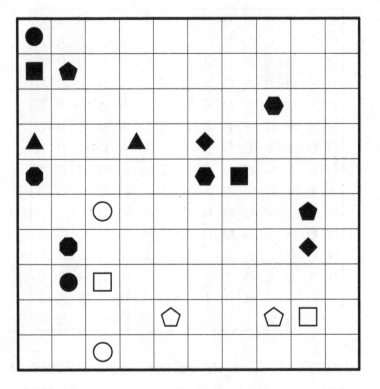

Slitherlink

Connect some of the dots to create a single loop, so that each
digit has the specified number of adjacent line segments. Dots
can be joined only by horizontal or vertical lines, and each dot
can be used only once.

```
·   ·   ·   ·   ·   ·   ·   ·   ·   ·   ·   ·
     1                           2       2
·   ·   ·   ·   ·   ·   ·   ·   ·   ·   ·   ·
     1               1                   3
·   ·   ·   ·   ·   ·   ·   ·   ·   ·   ·   ·
  3  1     2      3      3  0
·   ·   ·   ·   ·   ·   ·   ·   ·   ·   ·   ·
  3  1     0      2      2       3
·   ·   ·   ·   ·   ·   ·   ·   ·   ·   ·   ·
     1     2  3  2
·   ·   ·   ·   ·   ·   ·   ·   ·   ·   ·   ·
              2  3  1       1
·   ·   ·   ·   ·   ·   ·   ·   ·   ·   ·   ·
   1     2     3     1      0  3
·   ·   ·   ·   ·   ·   ·   ·   ·   ·   ·   ·
     2  0     2      3      1  3
·   ·   ·   ·   ·   ·   ·   ·   ·   ·   ·   ·
   1           0           2
·   ·   ·   ·   ·   ·   ·   ·   ·   ·   ·   ·
   0     0                 2
·   ·   ·   ·   ·   ·   ·   ·   ·   ·   ·   ·
```

Session 43

Sudoku

Place a number from 1 to 9 into each empty square, so that no digit repeats in any row, column or bold-lined 3×3 box.

	5						1	
9	8						4	2
			1		8			
	7	9		6	2			
	9	4		2	1			
		7		4				
2	7						3	8
	3						5	

Touchy

Place a letter from A to H into each empty square in such a way that no letter repeats in any row or column. Additionally, identical letters may not be in diagonally touching squares.

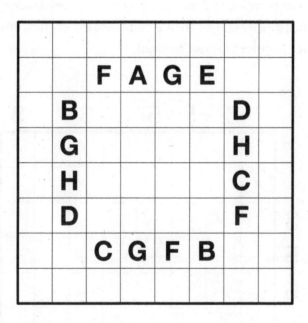

Train tracks

Draw track pieces in some squares to complete a single track
that travels all the way from its entrance in the leftmost column
to its exit in the bottom row. It can't otherwise exit the grid, nor
can it cross itself. Numbers outside the grid reveal the number
of track pieces in some rows and columns. Every track piece
must either go straight or turn a right-angled corner, and all
given track segments must be used.

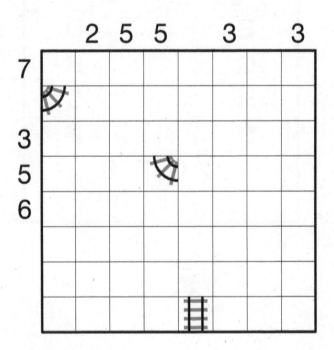

7. Plastic fantastic

Every few weeks – a bit longer if you're older – the cells in your skin get refreshed with new ones. Gut cells are also regenerated, new red blood cells are born. In fact, replacement of the body's cells with fresh ones is the norm.

Biologists had long regarded the brain as different: the adult brain was seen as non-renewable (no new neurons) and relatively resistant to change. However, this dogma crumbled in the 1960s in favour of a much more dynamic view of the brain, as an organ in a state of constant change. A new word began to circulate to reflect this revolution: 'neuroplasticity'.

This chapter is about neuroplasticity over the lifespan and how it explains brain resilience. We will look at these questions:

- What is neuroplasticity and why is it so important?
- How does it change over the course of our lives?
- What can taxi drivers, bilingual people, and musicians teach us about neuroplasticity?
- How do researchers think neuroplasticity works in the brain?
- What can all this tell us about doing puzzles?

Contrary to what we used to think, change in the adult brain is not just possible – it is a defining feature. Here's how.

What is neuroplasticity?

The 'plastic' in neuroplasticity means 'easy to mould or adapt'. Driven by genetics, your early years, and then what you are exposed to and get up to for the rest of your life, the structure and function of the brain are constantly changing and adapting, right up to the end. In response to learning and experiences, your brain is literally rewiring itself, all over the place, all the time. One of my favourite definitions of neuroplasticity is the 'subtle but orchestrated dance between the brain and the environment'.

Neuroplasticity, responding to learning and the environment, is what builds your young adult brain. It is why brain resilience is possible, because the brain is changed by experience. Neuroplasticity is why you can remember anything at all, learn to play the piano, or speak Spanish – it's at the heart of cognitive reserve. It is why doing puzzles regularly is good for your grey matter. It's behind rehabilitation after stroke and brain injury. (Neuroplasticity is also behind addiction, chronic pain, and post-traumatic stress disorder – but we won't dwell on those here.)

The term 'neuroplasticity' is itself used in a rather plastic way. At its broadest, neuroplasticity covers changes at multiple scales at different times: areas of the cerebral cortex take on new functions; nerves are formed or lost; new networks are created, strengthened or destroyed; nerve cells grow or lose branches;

and the synapses between cells are formed and strengthened, weakened or lost.

Neuroplasticity is thus a topic with many facets. We're going to look at it only through the lens of brain resilience and mental stimulation.[1]

To understand the role of neuroplasticity in brain resilience and puzzling, we will again need to take a life-course approach. This is because, although the brain retains plasticity at all ages, at some stages in life it is more plastic than others – so-called critical and sensitive periods. Let's see how.

Developmental neuroplasticity

Although neuroplasticity is lifelong, the brain is particularly malleable in its first few years. This is when newborn babies are exposed to the outside world of sights and sounds and smells, of things to touch and taste. During these early years children's brains are sculpted – so-called developmental neuroplasticity – to produce the overarching architecture. We'll come on to adult neuroplasticity shortly, which is about more detailed brain-sculpting.

At birth, a human baby's brain has about 100 billion neurons. By adulthood it will have lost about 15 per cent and be left with

---

1   If you're after uplifting stories about the role of neuroplasticity in rehabilitation or the latest in applied medical research, there are some great books out there. Norman Doidge's *The Brain That Changes Itself: Stories of Personal Triumph from the Frontiers of Brain Science* (Penguin, 2007), for example, is an enjoyable and accessible read.

'only' 86 billion. Synapses follow an even more dramatic culling, known as 'synaptic pruning'. At birth the neurons are relatively poorly connected, but the infant's brain makes synapses in the cortex like they're going out of fashion. They peak at around two years but their number will have fallen by half by the time the brain is mature.

What happens during this developmental sculpting is that the young brain starts out deliberately overwired. Then – through a combination of genetics and exposure to the environment – excess material is removed. The arbiter of what stays and what goes is brutal: if it isn't used, it's removed.

As children are exposed to sensory information, as they learn and grow, the networks, nerves, and synapses that get used and stimulated get strengthened and become more active. Like footpaths across a field, those that are not used become weaker and lost. 'Pruning' is a good analogy because the brain is winnowing out what it does not need – what is not used – and allocating more resource to what it does. What remains is stronger, less becomes more.

If that feels ruthlessly Darwinian, that's because it is, at different levels: neurons are competing for cortical real estate (see an example later in this chapter) and natural selection has favoured babies whose brains have developmental plasticity. Their owners have the best chance of growing up in a complex world to pass on their genes.

The visual pathway provides some good examples of developmental neuroplasticity tied to certain sensitive periods. If a child is born with a cataract in one eye and this goes uncorrected, the developing visual pathway from that eye is not stimulated. The pathway is not built as strongly, and the child will have permanently damaged sight from that eye. The unaffected eye, like an animal moving into unoccupied territory, extends its footprint in the visual cortex to include the spare area.

What happens in children who are born blind and learn to read Braille is even more dramatic. First they develop incredibly sensitive fingertips. Then the signals from the fingertips get rerouted to the visual cortex, which would be 'expecting' to receive a signal from the eyes but is not getting that. Instead, the visual cortex processes the signals from the fingers *as if they had come from the eyes*. The visual cortex is able to work out shapes (for example), without caring which 'input device' (i.e. the eye or fingertip) is sending it information.

Neuroplasticity is greatest in our early years, which is why formal education weighs so heavy on the scales of brain resilience. But there is also a second, smaller phase of developmental neuroplasticity around early adulthood. This second overgrow-and-prune-back strategy – again, what is not used is lost – starts before puberty and lasts until our early twenties. But this time it happens mainly in the prefrontal cortex.

Recall how this part of the brain is important for rational thought, decision-making, control of impulses, and risk assessment. As adolescents begin to think and act like adults, this is reflected in the synaptic pruning of their prefrontal cortex. Adolescence is also a time when axons get more myelinated and hence carry signals faster. These changes make the developing teenage brain less able to work at times – imagine living in a house that is being rewired and still expecting all the sockets to be fine. So, if you're a despairing parent, spare a thought for the state of your adolescent's plastic brain before you comment on the state of their bedroom.

Adult neuroplasticity

If you're past twenty-five and wondering about your brain now, what about neuroplasticity in adults? This includes those stories of dramatic rehabilitation, such as recovery from brain trauma. On a more everyday level, adult neuroplasticity in the mature brain enables learning, memory, and proper functioning. It also helps us to get better at puzzles, and thus hopefully stave off cognitive decline and dementia.

Adult neuroplasticity is not as dramatic as the developmental version, because the coarse architecture of the brain has already been set out. But, as we'll see, there is still huge potential for change in the adult brain. This is why resilience can still be built long after the brain is mature. Neuroplastic changes such as the birth of new neurons and new synapses lessen as we mature and age, but they continue right up to death. Again, natural selection has favoured adult brains that have been well sculpted but retain just the right amount of plasticity to adapt to an unpredictable environment. Let's look at some everyday case studies.

One of the most famous examples of everyday adult neuroplasticity is licensed London black-cab drivers. London cabbies are, uniquely and even in the age of the sat-nav,[2] still

---

2   Using GPS for navigation makes you worse at spatial learning. If you don't use it, you lose it!

required to memorise over 300 different routes and all their roads across the city's 25,000 streets. This learning is known as 'the Knowledge'. It generally necessitates three hours of study every day for four years, rote learning from maps. People also do practice runs on a moped.

Researchers used structural MRI to scan cabbies' brains and compared them with the brains of London bus drivers, who drive the same roads but on a small set of fixed routes. They found something startling. The backs of the taxi drivers' hippocampi, parts of the brain used to store spatial memories,[3] were larger than in the bus drivers.

The longer the taxi drivers had been working the bigger the change, so it seemed that using 'the Knowledge' was causing the increase – it's not the case that people with naturally large hippocampi and good spatial memory are somehow driven towards a career in the cab. And when the cabbies retired, their hippocampi began to shrink back to normal size.

How is such neuroplasticity linked to our story of brain resilience? We saw above how resilience to cognitive ageing or dementia was linked to challenging yourself regularly with puzzles. A 2015 study looked at more than 300 healthy adults aged forty-three to seventy-three. Those who regularly played cards or draughts or who did crosswords or other puzzles had

---

3 Damage to the hippocampus in people with Alzheimer's disease can cause them to get lost in familiar places. Their memory for spaces is being degraded.

better scores on tests of speed of reasoning and memory. More than that: they also had higher grey-matter volume in several places in their brains, including those that are particularly vulnerable to Alzheimer's pathology such as the hippocampus. So, that could explain their brain resilience. We'll see below *how* neuroplasticity causes such changes in the brain.

Let's revisit those other well-studied activities that build brain resilience: speaking a second language and learning to play a musical instrument. What's going on in the brains of bilinguals and bassoonists?

When we looked at word puzzles (Chapter 4), we saw how there is a language network in the brain. This includes Broca's and Wernicke's areas, but also other regions in the left frontal, temporal, and parietal lobes. This network is in turn connected to the auditory and visual systems for language that is heard or read. These areas are all connected up by white-matter fibres so that they can 'talk' to each other. So, it turns out that language involves almost every region of the brain.

Structural brain scans show that the brains of active older bilingual people have more grey matter than those of matched monolingual people. Areas that are bulkier include parts of both the prefrontal and temporal lobes, as well as the hippocampus. Older bilingual people also have healthier white matter in the fibres that connect these regions. On non-linguistic tests of executive function, such as switching attention, older bilingual people out-performed older monolingual people. Their brains also work more efficiently in the prefrontal cortex and parts of the language network.

So, whether you look at brain structure or function, active bilingualism seems to be particularly good for the prefrontal cortex. This is exactly what you would predict from the hypothesis on brain resilience in this group, which states that actively bilingual people have to use extra attention to focus on just one language at once. (Otherwise you get intrusions from one language into the other.) The other challenge of bilingualism that builds up brain resilience is switching seamlessly between languages when the need arises. That is the kind of dynamic decision-making and control that is at the heart of executive function.

What about music? If you play an instrument well, you may underestimate how much is going on in your brain. A lot of what once needed to be thought about and learned becomes embedded and embodied.[4] To unpack just some of what's going on, when you play an instrument you are constantly adapting your touch, mapping your hand movements across it with the sounds you're making, and using higher-order cognition like memory, attention, and processing (if you're reading music). And that's without bringing in your emotional connection to the piece or the reward of playing it well.

Studies of musicians' brains reveal a lot of changes. Among the most prominent is increased grey matter in the auditory cortex of the temporal lobe close to Wernicke's area, where sound is processed, in the frontal lobe executive-function areas (to

---

4   We sometimes refer to muscle memory for actions that have become subconscious through practice. Sure, the muscles do their stuff at the end, but your memory for the procedure is firmly in the brain.

maintain overall control of playing), and in the hippocampus for memory. Musicians also have healthier white matter to make better connections between regions linked to sensory processing and fine motor skills.

One of the most obvious changes in the musical brain is in the primary motor cortex, a strip along the back of the frontal lobe. This controls voluntary muscle movement.[5] In musicians there is often an enlarged fold in the shape of the Greek letter omega (Ω) on the motor cortex, specifically the part that controls hand and finger movements. This raised area of grey matter is known as an 'omega sign' – or 'hand knob' for the less classically inclined. The omega sign appears on both sides of the brain in pianists but on only one side in violinists, linked to the finger (i.e. non-bow) hand that makes the notes. This story of repeat use causing brain growth really is just like a weightlifter's muscles.

For all these differences in the musical brain, the extent of the change is related to usage: playing for longer and practising more make for bigger changes. As with the taxi drivers and bilingual people, this suggests that musical training is mostly driving the effects – it's not that people get into playing because they have a predisposition to Brahms in their brains.

One thing does come across loud and clear from these examples. The people who showed most gains were the regular

5   The layout of the primary motor cortex, amazingly, is 'topographical': the order on the brain surface follows the body's own physical layout. So, along the strip of motor cortex in the brain run side by side the areas for shoulder, elbow, wrist, hand, and then the fingers, ending with the thumb.

puzzlers, the cabbies who studied over several years, the bilingual people who were the most proficient in their second language, and the experienced musicians with thousands of hours of practice behind them. So, the 'use' part of 'Use it or lose it' can involve a lot of effort.

On the social activities linked to brain resilience, which you will recall included religion, I stumbled on a study in which practising Catholics and atheists (as controls) considered fully forty-eight ethical conundrums while inside a functional MRI scanner. The title tells you all need to know: 'Roman Catholic beliefs produce characteristic neural responses to moral dilemmas'. The much-ridiculed phrenologists included an 'organ of religious veneration' in the brain as early as 1815, so maybe they were on to something after all.[6]

Let's pause to pull a few strands together.

We saw earlier how cognitively and socially stimulating activities such as regularly doing puzzles, being bilingual, or learning to play an instrument increase brain resilience. (Don't forget the benefits of *physical* exercise for brain resilience too.) We've just seen evidence of the kinds of neuroplastic changes in the brain that some of this learning and mental activity generates.

Did you notice how the regions of the brain that show the most growth in grey-matter volume and functional activity in

---

6   Phrenology was from soon after its birth derided as 'bumpology' and
    it never had a strong evidence base, even by the different standards of
    its time. Yet its largely correct idea of cerebral localisation stole a
    march on Broca and Wernicke (see Chapter 2) by fifty years.

high-brain-resilience groups overlap with the regions of the brain that deteriorate most quickly in age-related cognitive decline and many dementias? These include the prefrontal cortex, the hippocampus, and regions of white matter.

That supports the whole resilience theory. But how does it work? How does cognitive or social stimulation cause the changes in nerves and networks that give us brain resilience? Let's summarise what we know.

Neuroplasticity and brain resilience

We've seen how *structural* changes are thought to underlie brain reserve and how *functional* changes are thought to underlie cognitive reserve. But not how each is built up – how cognitive, social, and physical activity build brain resilience. We don't know the answers for sure, but we have some ideas.

Basis of brain reserve

One of the most exciting recent discoveries, and one of the current hot and most hotly debated topics in neuroplasticity, is adult neurogenesis.

Recall how neuroplasticity falls with age, and that the adult brain is less plastic than the developing neonatal and infant brain. Up until the 1990s, mainstream science said that neurogenesis – the formation of new nerve cells – simply did not happen at all in the adult human brain. It's a controversial topic, and the evidence is stronger in other mammals, but many neuroscientists now accept that new nerve cells *are* formed in several places in the mature human brain. The evidence for adult neurogenesis is strongest at sites within the hippocampi and the lateral ventricles (fluid-filled cavities), and weaker at other sites including the amygdala (the emotional processing centre, next to the hippocampus). Neurogenesis is thought to continue in healthy older people right up until death, although it's very much reduced in people with diseases such as Alzheimer's.

As these newborn neurons mature, they migrate and are incorporated into the existing neural network of the hippocampus. Here they form new synapses and act to support – rather than disrupt – learning and memory. (That's a bit like grafting a new arm on to a juggler without dropping any balls.)

In rodents, the birth of new nerve cells is stimulated by regular physical activity on a treadmill, but many of those neurons are destined to die. It is environmental enrichment – ratty toys and mousey objects that are changed often – that helps the neurons to survive, mature, and integrate. While it's more certain in rodents, there is some evidence that human hippocampal neurogenesis follows the same rules. So, to birth these neurons and then keep them alive we need to be physically as well as mentally and socially active. Exercise of either body or mind alone is not enough.

Neurogenesis thus offers one way that cognitive stimulation might build brain reserve: hippocampal volume increases in cognitively and physically active adults as new nerve cells get incorporated into it.

Staying at the structural level and with a bit more certainty, changes to the shape of existing neurons are also thought to underlie increased grey-matter volume and increased brain reserve. These changes include more branching of dendrons and greater numbers of spines, as well as more branching of axons at their terminals. Synapses are formed where dendritic spines meet axon terminals, so these changes make for more synapses.

New spines and synapses rely on neuronal gene expression and are part of the later stages of memory consolidation and learning. Stronger neural networks have more axon terminals, more spines, and more synapses. In rats, at least, these kinds of changes are seen when the rodents are stimulated with a varied and changing environment.

Finally, there are the observed structural changes in white matter in groups with higher brain reserve, which is likely to reflect thicker or healthier myelin sheaths. You've seen how important white matter is for long-range transmission of signals, so white matter that is less prone to degradation in age-related cognitive decline or dementia should lead to better brain resilience.

There are a couple of other ways that regions of the brain might increase in resilience but that don't involve nerve tissue directly: angiogenesis and glial cells. Angiogenesis is when new blood vessels grow from existing vessels into a region, which leads to greater brain tissue volume. The new blood vessels bring in extra oxygen and glucose, and so support greater nerve activity.

Glial cells, those Best Supporting Actors at the brain's Oscars, are hugely important in helping neurons work and they're present in about equal numbers in the adult brain. Different types of glial cell create the myelin sheath, hoover up cell debris, promote neuroplasticity, and modify how signals are transmitted at synapses. It's thought they might become larger or more numerous in active areas of the brain, leading to an increase in tissue volume.

Basis of cognitive reserve

Let's turn from structural to functional effects: changes in the efficiency of neural networks or new pathways that are brought into play (active cognitive reserve). The mechanisms here are all assumed to be at the level of the synapse. That means changes to how existing synapses – and hence pathways – work.

Recall how at the synapse, the electrical signal is carried across the gap by a chemical neurotransmitter. Once the neurotransmitter has crossed the gap it binds to a specific molecular receptor – like a key fitting a lock – on the other side to carry the signal to the next neuron and so on its way as a new electrical impulse.

Now, if a neuron persistently excites a downstream nerve cell by sending repeated signals over a short enough period, then the first neuron becomes more efficient at firing the second. This means that the connection (synapse) between the two is strengthened, so if the first neuron later fires again, then the synapse is more effective. There is a lot of evidence that such changes are the basis of learning and long-term memory. Recall how neurons that are strongly linked by repeat activation become associated into a network such as a memory trace.

This process of synaptic plasticity has its own catch phrase that we saw before: 'Neurons that fire together wire together.' But the same principle also lies behind more familiar phrases, such as 'Practice makes perfect' and – as we've learned to chant in our sleep by now – 'Use it or lose it'.

We know a lot about how synapses are strengthened by repeat stimulation, but feel free to skip this biochemical detail if you want to. One thing that happens is that the receptors 'waiting' for the neurotransmitter on the dendritic spine get chemically modified. This makes the receptor more sensitive to the neurotransmitter – the 'lock' (receptor) is 'oiled' and so is opened by the 'key' (neurotransmitter) more easily. On top of this, extra receptors that the neuron has been holding in reserve (so, not made anew) are moved up to the post-synaptic membrane. These changes mean that, when the upstream nerve later fires, the synapse generates a much stronger response and the network that it is part of will light up. 'Memories Are Made of This'. Do note that a stable long-term memory also requires subsequent anatomical changes in the synapse, driven by gene expression and protein synthesis (as outlined previously).

In addition to active synapses becoming more efficient, functional neuroplasticity can also be caused by activation of 'silent' synapses. This is a bit like opening up a stretch of road that has been closed for a while and, like that, could allow for the nerve impulse to take a different route. Activation of silent synapses is thought to be one of the ways that active cognitive reserve works, when new networks are recruited to compensate for disease or injury that has damaged the usual routes.

Engines of neuroplasticity

Those are some of the likely causes of the changes seen in the brains of cognitively and socially active people with high brain resilience. Which of the above mechanisms are most important, under what circumstances, where, and in whom has yet to be discovered. The evidence is evolving – adult neurogenesis in particular is controversial – so expect a complicated picture.

Complexity aside, an overarching theme does emerge: in a range of settings, doing mentally stimulating activities or having an enriched environment promotes all the above changes (as does physical exercise). The evidence for this is much stronger in rodents than in humans, but even in us the same kinds of rule seem to apply.

In short, the engines of neuroplastic change as far as the environment goes – because you're not going to change your genes – are variety, stimulation, and challenge. Doing new things creates new connections, new networks. Repeat exercise makes these connections and networks stronger.

You should briefly meet one of the star molecules in all this, because it has an almost magical effect on the brain: brain-derived neurotrophic factor (BDNF). BDNF is made naturally in the brain and found mainly in the cerebral cortex and hippocampus. It is central to neuroplasticity, memory, and learning.

One of the ways BDNF works its magic is by promoting neurogenesis. BDNF is why physical exercise is able to offset the very gradual shrinkage of the hippocampus that comes with normal ageing (see Chapter 3). It is thought that exercise causes us to make lots of BDNF in the brain, which in turn leads to neurogenesis in the hippocampus. Exercise has been best studied here, but there is early evidence that cognitively stimulating activities and even mindfulness could raise BDNF concentrations in healthy older adults too.

But BDNF doesn't just help to make new neurons: it also keeps existing ones healthy, promotes myelination, supports the formation of synapses, and helps to form memories. It is no surprise that BDNF has been called, keeping to the horticultural metaphors, 'fertiliser for the brain'.

So, as we come almost to the end of *Mind Games*, what have we learned – what fruit have we harvested?

Ours has been a twisty old journey on hugely different scales, from global demographic changes in our ageing society to molecular changes in our ageing – but still plastic – neurons. I hope it's been clear how you (and I) fit in, whether that's on this scale looking 'up' to community or 'down' to the cell. Where we fit matters, because we all have agency in this. Our attitudes and actions shape how we respond to ageing in ourselves and others, with or without the conditions like dementia that Alzheimer's Society is so passionate about. And our attitudes and actions massively shape how well we will all age, whether in an active, healthy way or less so. We really are all in this together.

As part of helping you to keep mentally active the puzzles have – I hope – been fun. But they have as often as not been a Trojan Horse for this wider agenda. For 'The Times They Are a-Changin'', and not just for that Woodstock generation. It's for all of us to decide how.

8. About Alzheimer's Society

At Alzheimer's Society, we know that dementia devastates lives. That's why, as the UK's leading dementia charity, we're a vital source of support for everyone living with dementia today. We're also a powerful force for change, campaigning to make dementia the priority it should be and funding groundbreaking research.

Dementia is the biggest health and social challenge of our time. There are currently estimated to be 900,000 people in the UK with dementia. Many are undiagnosed and facing the realities of their condition alone. With the help of our supporters, Alzheimer's Society is changing that. We're made up of people with dementia, carers, trusted experts, campaigners, researchers, and clinicians. We are the UK's largest collective force of people with unparalleled knowledge and over forty years of experience addressing the biggest challenges facing people living with dementia.

Through donations, we provide a vital support line, online and print information and advice, and expert dementia advisers. We also have an online community. All this means that people living with dementia can get the practical guidance they need to make it through the hardest and most frightening times of their lives. Donations from our supporters and fundraisers mean we can help those who need it most, and that whatever people are going through they can turn to us for help.

As well as the vital help we provide, we bring hope. We know that research is key if we want to change the landscape of dementia in the future. That's why, right now, we're backing the world's brightest minds and funding over 600 research projects to find the best ways to get early diagnosis, innovate care, and develop targeted treatments.

One in three people born in the UK today will develop dementia in their lifetime. We don't want anyone to face the realities of dementia alone. That's why we need all the backing we can get.

With your help we can give vital support to those who need it most, hold decision makers to account, and fund groundbreaking research to transform the future for everyone living with dementia.

If you're able to support us, fundraise for us, partner with us, or campaign alongside us visit **alzheimers.org.uk**.

If you're living with dementia and need practical advice, emotional support, or guidance, we're here for you. Call us today on **0333 150 3456**.

Enjoyed *Mind Games*?

Continue to keep your brain active with Alzheimer's Society's monthly *Brain Workout* puzzles delivered straight to your door.

Brain Workout is a fun way to keep your brain active while also supporting those living with dementia. If you sign up, you can choose how much you wish to give on a monthly basis and in return you'll receive a pack of mind-stimulating puzzles straight to your door every month! With a different set of puzzles in every pack like cryptic crosswords or tricky number puzzles, there's plenty to keep your brain on its toes, all while supporting a vital cause.

Your donation will go towards improving the lives of those affected by dementia, from funding lifeline services to supporting world-leading research. Visit **alzheimers.org.uk/ brainworkout** to find out more.

Appendix 1

A puzzle routine

You can work through the puzzles in *Mind Games* in any order you like and at any pace. We're all different in how quickly we complete puzzles: some people will zip through a crossword over a cheeky cappuccino but others will get through a whole pot of tea. We also differ in how quickly each of us might take to complete one type of puzzle compared with another. (As a writer, I'm much happier with the verbal than the visuospatial ones.)

That said, here are some general suggestions about how you might maximise the benefits of puzzling for your grey matter. Please treat these as 'informed common sense' rather than based on a rigorous research evidence base: there isn't one.

1. If it fits the spare time you have, go for 'little and often' rather than be a 'weekend (puzzle) warrior'. Either fit a bit of puzzling into your routine every day or maybe have three (non-consecutive) puzzle days spread over the week. If you struggle to fit around either of those, any puzzling you can squeeze in at any time is going to be better than none at all.

2. 'How long should I commit to puzzles each day?' is commonly asked and is what philosophers should call a 'piece of string' question: how long have you got? In practice, many people find between 10 and 30 minutes a

day is about right – maybe 10–15 minutes if you're doing a *daily* brain workout and 30 minutes if you're puzzling *every other* day. Any of these should give you long enough to get your brain firmly into puzzle mode but not so long that you lose focus and motivation, which are both vital.

3. When you're doing the puzzles, try to keep to the order of sessions as set out in the book. As you'll see, they start with the easier puzzles and gradually get harder. Following the sessions as set out means you're learning and challenging yourself as you go, the same as if you were gradually learning a more complex piece of music or the future perfect tense in German.

4. The sessions are set out so that each one might take you about 20–40 minutes, but that is only a very rough guide, not a target or limit. You will notice that the later, more difficult, sessions tend to include fewer puzzles, so you have longer for each. If you need more time, or you need a break to let your mind wander, that's fine. (How often has the solution to a tricky problem just popped into your mind when you were thinking of something else entirely?)

5. You might find that you're quicker doing some types of puzzles than others, either through familiarity or just how your mind seems to work. That might tempt you to jump ahead to harder puzzles of a type you're familiar with and hence skip over puzzles of a different type. That's fine, but you might then come back to the puzzles you find harder later. You'll gain more from the effort and new learning they will require, and you do need to work out different parts of the grey matter, which means different puzzle types. Maybe view doing the ones you find easier as a 'reward' for grafting over those you find a bit harder. No pain, no gain!

6. Above all, have fun! You'll stay motivated if you enjoy the
   puzzles, and those dopamine hits you get from the right
   answer will help you learn and get better. And remember
   the benefits of social activity: why not share a puzzle with
   a friend, or work on one together?

	Example Puzzle Routine		
	Every day (10–15 minutes)	Every other day (or so) (30 minutes)	'Any time I get a spare moment to myself'
Day 1	Session 1 (start)	Session 1	Try to follow sessions sequentially, noting the caveats above
Day 2	Session 1 (end)	–	
Day 3	Session 2 (start)	Session 2	
Day 4	Session 2 (end)	–	
Day 5	Session 3 (start)	Session 3	
Day 6	Session 3 (end)	–	
Day 7	Session 4 (start)	Session 4	
And so on . . .			

Finally, one thing you've learned from the book is that good
brain health over the lifespan requires a lot more than just
regular mental stimulation. Turn the page to Appendix 2 for a
summary of how else you can keep the grey matter happy.

Appendix 2

Healthy brain ageing: the other pieces of the jigsaw

You've seen how puzzles and other forms of mental or social stimulation can help to keep your brain trim, but there are lots of other ways too, and you're best off trying a wide range of approaches.[1] Following all the recommendations presented here, together with lifelong cognitive and social stimulation, could prevent or delay a massive 40 per cent of all dementia.

But first, a note of caution: the following is general information for healthy people, and should not be considered medical advice. If a qualified professional suggests you do differently from any of these tips, you should follow them, not me.

Healthy heart, healthy head

We saw in Chapter 3 that poor cardiovascular health is a risk factor for brain diseases such as stroke, Alzheimer's and vascular dementia – and hence why 'What's good for the heart is good for the head' is true. Let's unpack that a bit.

---

1   The Global Council on Brain Health website (Google it) pulls all this together in a very accessible and action-based way.

Manage health conditions

For good cardiovascular health, try to keep to a healthy weight[2] and to avoid getting high blood pressure, high cholesterol, or type 2 diabetes if you can. If you do develop any of those conditions, keeping it under control by following medical advice will help to lower your stroke and dementia risk. To reduce your chances of getting them in the first place, physical exercise is important (see below), as is eating a healthy balanced diet and not smoking. Let's look at those last two in a bit more detail.

Eat well

Two diets are much touted as good for the brain: the Dietary Approaches to Stop Hypertension (DASH) diet and the Mediterranean diet. They seem to work mainly by promoting good cardiovascular health and a healthy weight, but the antioxidants in the fruit and veg they recommend also reduce damaging inflammation.

In practice, the DASH and Mediterranean diets are similar and less radical than you might be wondering. Expect to eat more plants (vegetables, fruits, grains, nuts, and seeds) and low-fat

---

2   It's in mid-life that obesity and high blood pressure are risk factors for dementia. You often see body mass index (weight in kilograms divided by height in metres squared) discussed with values of $18.5-24.9$ kg/m² considered healthy and those over 30 kg/m² considered obese for most adults. But excess fat around the abdomen is the real problem, and so the ratio of waist to height is another measure of obesity.

dairy, and to get most animal protein from eggs, fish, and poultry, with less red – and especially processed – meat.

Most adults who are not pregnant don't need supplements, so take one only if advised to by a doctor.

Don't smoke

You know this, but smoking is bad for you in lots of ways, including increasing your risk of dementia and stroke. Cigarette smoke is a cocktail of nasties that damage blood vessels and cause inflammation. If you smoke and are able to quit, your risk of dementia and stroke falls at any age. Vaping is better than smoking tobacco because then you don't get the tar. Switching to nothing if you can is better still. Ask your GP or pharmacist for help.

Protect your head

There is growing recognition of how much harm blows to the head can cause. We've known about punch-drunk boxers for a century, but the latest research is about repeated head trauma without knockouts as a risk factor for dementia. Sport is still in the spotlight: bruising tackles in rugby, clashes of heads in soccer – possibly even just too many headers. How blunt head trauma causes dementia is not clear, and the evidence is still emerging, but phosphorylated tau protein is again in the dock.

As important as it is to stay physically active, when exercising it's equally important to protect your head: wear a helmet when cycling, skateboarding, or horse-riding, and follow sports concussion protocols. And watch out for developments in this fast-moving area.

'Be not solitary, be not idle'[3]

This section covers activities that work by lowering the chance of getting brain disease in the first place (like all those above) and also by increasing brain resilience if you do get dementia or stroke. So, they have a dual action.

Be physically active

If you were unwise enough to choose just one thing to keep your grey matter happy, regular physical activity would be a better choice than puzzling. Why? Because moving your body is good for your brain at any age and in lots of different ways. Physical activity makes for better sleep, helps with weight and depression, lowers blood pressure and diabetes risk, and promotes blood vessel and heart health. Via all these effects, it is also helping to prevent Alzheimer's, vascular dementia, and stroke.

On the neuron level, regular physical activity reverses the normal shrinkage of the hippocampus that starts from age sixty. That's down to BDNF, increased synapse creation, reduced inflammation, and formation of new blood vessels (Chapter 7). Physical activity is great for neuroplasticity.

----

3   This advice is from Robert Burton's *The Anatomy of Melancholy* (1621). Four centuries on, parts of it feel refreshingly current.

What kind of exercise is best? Aim for 150 minutes across the week of aerobic activity (brisk walking, cycling, etc) and mix in a couple of days a week when you do strength training (weights or squats, for example). Good news if you're more couch potato than gym bunny: the biggest benefits come from just getting off the sofa to do a bit, rather than in pushing it to extremes.

Sleep well

The importance of sleep for brain health is a pretty hot topic.[4] Sleep is really important for consolidation of learning and memory. As we snooze, our neurons replay their waking activity and remodel neural pathways and synapses. Sleep promotes synaptic plasticity and good cognitive ageing. Furthermore, harmful β-amyloid is cleared while we sleep.

How much shut-eye should you get? The current consensus is seven to eight hours sleep a night – too little sleep is almost certainly bad for you and too much might be as well, although the jury on that is still out. If you struggle with sleep, check out the Global Council on Brain Health website for tips. Advice on sleep routines tends to come packaged as 'sleep hygiene', so look out for that phrase.

---

4   Matthew Walker's *Why We Sleep: The New Science of Sleep and Dreams* (Penguin, 2018) makes for good bedtime reading. You'll learn how poor-quality sleep is also a risk factor for obesity, type 2 diabetes, heart disease, and stroke.

Limit your alcohol intake

The evidence on alcohol is really messy, but most experts agree that a small amount reduces dementia risk. *How* small is the rub: some studies would let you drink as much as fourteen UK units a week – about six pints of beer or six medium glasses of wine – before your dementia risk rises but in others it's much less. Wine with every evening meal can easily push you over that limit. What is not disputed is that alcohol in large amounts is toxic to nerve cells, causing inflammation and vitamin B1 deficiency.

Regularly downing more than the NHS-recommended safe levels of alcohol increases your risk of dementia and other conditions such as high blood pressure, stroke, heart attack, type 2 diabetes, and obesity. So, good brain health means keeping a close eye on how much alcohol you're drinking. And if you're not a drinker, don't start now to reduce your dementia risk.

Look after your mental health

Long-term stress and depression are both probable risk factors for cognitive ageing and dementia. They seem to work partly through hormones such as cortisol, which is linked to loss of grey and white matter and increased β-amyloid. Talk to your GP to get help with managing stress and depression.

Get your hearing checked

Mid-life hearing impairment is a more recent addition to dementia risk factors, with evidence still coming in. It may be that hearing loss harms the grey matter because there is less stimulation. Or perhaps dealing with the consequences of hearing loss pulls brain resources away from other tasks. If so, hearing loss could act mainly to reduce brain resilience. If you're struggling to follow conversations or you have the TV or radio volume cranked up, then get your hearing checked out.[5] If you're younger, try not to expose yourself to excessive noise for long periods.

5   Alzheimer's Society is working with eargym (**www.eargym.world**) to support people affected by dementia to care for their hearing before the need for hearing aids.

Appendix 3

Computerised brain training: hope or hype?

Dementia is now the most-feared disease among the over fifties. One market response to this has been commercial training programs, games, or apps: the likes of Lumosity, BrainGymmer, and BrainHQ. Usually referred to as 'brain training',[1] these programs are sold on a promise that they will make you smarter and prevent cognitive decline. And sold at scale too: the brain-training industry worldwide is set to be worth US$17.5 billion by 2025. Big money, but does brain training work?

This is how the programs are meant to work, according to their developers. A program – often in the form of a game – guides you through a set of tasks, each designed to target specific cognitive domains (attention, working memory, processing speed, etc). You get feedback and encouragement, so the program is fun and motivating. The tasks are repeated and get more challenging, such that over time you are meant to

---

1   The terminology here is not used consistently, but it can be helpful to distinguish between computerised, self-directed brain training (as outlined here) and cognitive training. The latter seeks to maintain or improve a specific, targeted cognitive function via structured, guided practice done individually or in a group. This has not stopped some people calling brain training 'computerised cognitive training'.

strengthen that cognitive ability – recall our principles in Chapter 4. That beefed-up cognitive skill then translates into real-world benefits, including a slower rate of cognitive ageing or better everyday skills. That is not intuitively bad science. What's not to like?

The issue is that the programs simply might not deliver on those bold claims. The big controversy with brain training has always been whether getting better at a task *in the program* translates into anything meaningful in the real world, away from the screen. The marketing blurbs promise big: you will stay sharp, think fast, improve your short-term memory, focus better, and remember more – in short, you'll be combatting age-related cognitive decline. Some games even claimed to help you prevent dementia – or did before the regulators put an end to that.

There is a lot at stake here, not just a huge commercial interest. If the games were proven to offer real-world benefits – possibly even slower cognitive ageing – that would be economic and medical manna. But if they do not provide these benefits, worried consumers keen to do something positive for their brain health could be wasting time and money that could be better spent on something else.

This controversy has led to combative statements from both scientists and the industry, and at least one US court case. What does the latest evidence say? A lot of studies have been done, but not all of them have been of high quality. One thing to put to bed first. There is no reliable evidence that any brain-training program reduces dementia risk or improves cognition in anyone who already has dementia or mild cognitive impairment – but there is a need for more and better research in this group. Everything that follows is about cognitively healthy older people.

To give the brain-training programs a fair hearing it's helpful to break the claims down. First the boring bit that no one disputes: if you train on a task in the program, you will get better at that *same* task in the program. Practice makes perfect.

Broadening out a bit, does training on one cognitive domain make you better at different tasks that use the same domain (known as 'near transfer')? For example, would a program that trained your working memory lead to better scores in tests of working memory outside the program? A 2020 paper that combined results from more than forty studies showed that near transfer was seen for some cognitive domains after use of brain-training programs – notably processing speed and working memory. Fewer studies report near transfer in attention and executive function, such as reasoning and decision-making.

Finally, the billion-dollar questions of 'far transfer': do brain-training programs lead to any improvements in cognitive domains that were not part of the program, and do these gains convert into benefits in daily function? That 2020 paper found small but significant transfer to some untrained-for cognitive domains for healthy over sixties, but with a catch. Regular brain training in this group led to small but significant *perceived* improvements in processing speed and, with weaker evidence, in executive function, working memory, and possibly attention, even when these were not part of the training program. Training also led to small but significant improvements in *perceived*

everyday functioning – self-reported measures of mood and
wellbeing, and perceived cognitive functioning.

'Perceived' and 'self-reported' matter here: people felt they had
improved in all these areas, when they actually had not. ('Did
brain training work? Well, I *felt* it did.') But remember how
attitudes to your own brain health, abilities, and general positivity
are so important (Chapter 1)? The step from better self-
perception and mood to actual brain health gains could be small.

Where any degree of transfer has been proven, this seems to be
mostly for domains that are known to decline in healthy ageing,
such as processing speed and working memory. Any effects
were seen only over a few months at most. Only a few brain
training studies have looked at cognitive changes in the longer
term. It's also not clear if any one brain-training program is
better than any other.

Where does all that leave brain-training programs? Despite the
knockbacks, a multi-billion-dollar industry is not going away
soon. The latest research suggests some short-term benefits
beyond simply getting better at the game, but the gap between
these findings and the bold marketing claims still feels large.
More and better research is sorely needed, especially looking at
far transfer into measurable everyday functioning (shopping,
remembering people's names, managing medication) and
looking at gains beyond a few months. It may also be that the
benefits vary between people a lot, depending on their strengths
and weaknesses before training.

Should you invest in brain training? If you enjoy it and have the
time and money, then go ahead. Unless you have dementia, you

might get slightly better at some things and feel you've got better at others. As long as you're not playing for hours on end, the games aren't doing you any harm, and some studies even suggest you need thirty minutes each session to see any benefit. Just don't rely on brain-training programs as the main way to stimulate the brain – in fact, don't rely on any one thing.

Solutions

Sample puzzles

p. 72 Building blocks: B

p. 77 Add a word: AIR (AIRMAIL, AIRSTRIP, AIRSPACE, AIRLINE)

p. 81 Age puzzle: Amy is eighteen, Ben is thirty-two, and Claire is twenty-four.

p. 86 Brainteaser: Mr White was now matching Mr Green, who had started the day with a white tie. Mr White started with a grey tie, Mr Green with a white one, and Mr Grey with a green one.

Level 1: Warm-up puzzles

Session 1

p. 91 Cube counting: thirty-four cubes

p. 92 Anagrams: MAT, POSE, FOCUS, ASANA, POSTURE, BALANCE, BREATHING, MEDITATION

p. 93 Number chains: 21, 2, 34, 75

p. 94 Calcudoku:

⁴⁺⁴ 4	1	⁷⁺ 5	2	²⁻ 3
²⁺ 1	⁶⁺ 2	4	⁹⁰⁰ˣ 3	5
2	4	3	5	⁴⁺ 1
⁸⁺ 3	5	¹⁻ 2	1	4
5	³ˣ 3	1	²⁺ 4	2

Session 2

p. 97 Fold and punch: C

p. 97 Changed sets: NATO phonetic alphabet (TANGO, LIMA, KILO, BRAVO, GOLF)

p. 98 Number darts: $17 = 4 + 10 + 3$; $21 = 5 + 2 + 14$; $35 = 13 + 10 + 12$

p. 98 Complete the series: B (At each stage one extra side is added to the polygon, and one extra circle is added to the chain of circles on its perimeter. Odd-numbered chains of circles run clockwise from the top-centre of the polygon, while even-numbered chains of circles run anti-clockwise from the top-centre of the polygon.)

Session 3

p. 99 Hidden image: B

B

p. 99 Connected clues: Shakespearean characters (Orlando, Puck, Hamlet, Witches, Bottom)

p. 100 Number pyramid:

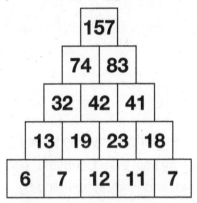

p. 101 Crack the code: d: RKJ (F = triangle points up; R = triangle points down; K = white triangle; G = black triangle; J = cross in top-right corner; L = cross in bottom-left corner)

Session 4

p. 102 Maze:

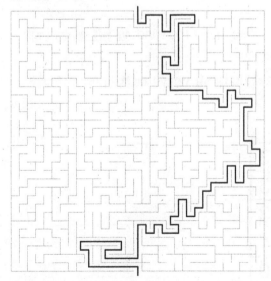

p. 103 Crossword:

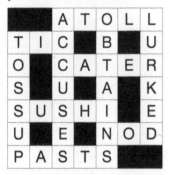

p. 104 Number teaser: fifteen flamingos and twenty-one swans

p. 104 Deductions: Peter is travelling by train from Denmark, Quinn is travelling by boat from Finland, and Rudy is travelling by bus from Austria.

Session 5

p. 105 Reflections: B

p. 105 Hidden words:

1 GREEN: According to legend, the o**gre en**vied the princess so much that he ate her.

2 WHITE: The woman who broke the windo**w hit e**very high note in her singing class.

3 SILVER: I don't use dried ba**sil ver**y much; I prefer to use fresh leaves.

p. 106 Dominoes:

2	1	3	3	0	3
2	3	0	0	4	3
0	1	0	1	4	3
2	1	4	2	4	1
2	1	4	4	2	0

Session 6

p. 107 Shape count: twenty-seven rectangles

p. 107 Start and end: O (OUTDO, ORZO, OVERDO, OREGANO)

p. 108 Futoshiki:

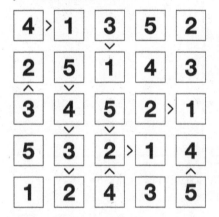

Session 7

p. 109 Top-down view: D

p. 110 Word circle: the word that includes all the letters is genius. Other words to find include genus, gin, gins, gnu, gnus, gun, guns, ins, sign, sin, sine, sing, singe, snug, suing, sun, sung, and using.

p. 110 Jigdoku:

C	B	D	E	A
E	A	B	C	D
B	D	C	A	E
A	C	E	D	B
D	E	A	B	C

Session 8

p. 111 Kakuro:

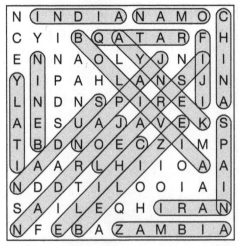

p. 112 Word ladder: one possible solution is LOW → LAW → JAW → JAR → BAR

p. 112 Tracing paper: A

Session 9

p. 113 Wordsearch:

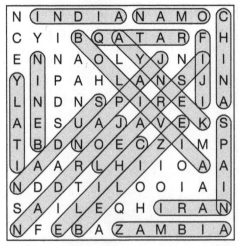

p. 114 Shapelink:

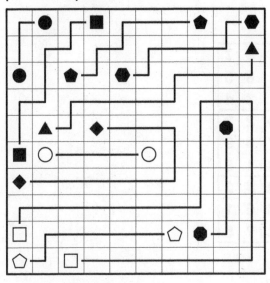

p. 115 Slitherlink:

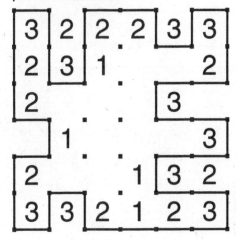

Session 10

p. 116 Sudoku:

8	2	5	1	3	4	6	9	7
9	4	3	2	6	7	1	8	5
7	6	1	5	8	9	2	3	4
6	7	4	9	1	8	5	2	3
5	1	8	3	4	2	7	6	9
3	9	2	6	7	5	4	1	8
1	8	6	7	5	3	9	4	2
2	3	7	4	9	6	8	5	1
4	5	9	8	2	1	3	7	6

p. 117 Touchy:

A	E	C	D	B	F
C	B	A	F	E	D
D	F	E	B	C	A
E	C	D	A	F	B
F	A	B	E	D	C
B	D	F	C	A	E

p. 118 Train tracks:

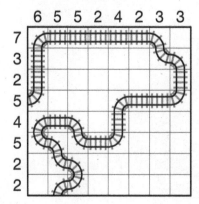

Level 2: Step-up puzzles

Session 11

p. 123 Building blocks: C

p. 123 Add a word: LAND (LANDLORD, LANDFILL, LANDSLIDE, LANDLOCKED)

p. 124 Age puzzle: Dom is fourteen, Eddie is eighteen, Frida is seven, and Greg is sixteen.

p. 124 Brainteaser: Paris > Madrid > Lisbon > Barcelona > Zurich > Prague > Berlin > Copenhagen

Session 12

p. 127 Cube counting: thirty-three cubes

p. 128 Anagrams: LION, ZEBRA, OKAPI, IMPALA, WARTHOG, GIRAFFE, ELEPHANT, RHINOCEROS

p. 129 Number chains: 14, 15, 21, 12

p. 130 Calcudoku:

5+		90×	6+	4×	12×
3	**2**	**6**	**5**	**1**	**4**
3÷					
2	**6**	**5**	**1**	**4**	**3**
10+			20×		3−
6	**1**	**3**	**4**	**5**	**2**
	2−		1÷	72×	
4	**3**	**1**	**2**	**6**	**5**
6+	9+	6+			
1	**5**	**4**	**3**	**2**	**6**
				3×	
5	**4**	**2**	**6**	**3**	**1**

Session 13

p. 133 Fold and punch: A

p. 133 Changed sets: associated with tennis (SERVE, RACKET, COURT, LAWN, LOVE)

p. 134 Number darts: 31 = 3 + 11 + 17; 48 = 15 + 8 + 25; 54 = 22 + 13 + 19

p. 134 Complete the series: C (At each stage the star appears in the position pointed to by the arrow in the previous box, in the colour [black or grey] indicated by that arrow. This means that you can use the boxes to the left and right of the empty square to work out the appearance of both the star [from the position and colour of the arrow in the box to the left] and the arrow [from the position and colour of the star in the box to its right].)

Session 14

p. 135 Hidden image: C

p. 135 Connected clues: Double 'Z' (drizzle, embezzle, blizzard, dazzle, buzzing)

p. 136 Number pyramid:

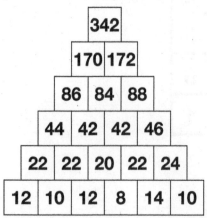

p. 137 Crack the code: c: DYZ (Q = flat hexagon top; D = pointed hexagon top; X = grey outer hexagon; Y = white outer hexagon; Z = small hexagon present; W = no small hexagon present)

Session 15

p. 138 Maze:

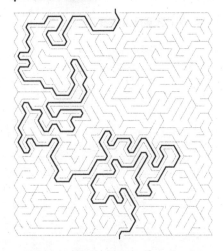

p. 139 Crossword:

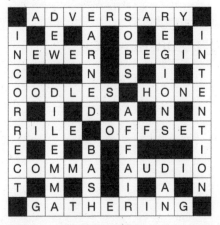

	A	D	V	E	R	S	A	R	Y	
I		E		A		O		E		I
N	E	W	E	R		B	E	G	I	N
C			N		S		I		T	
O	O	D	L	E	S		H	O	N	E
R		I		D		A		N		N
R	I	L	E		O	F	F	S	E	T
E		E		B		F				I
C	O	M	M	A		A	U	D	I	O
T		M		S		I		A		N
	G	A	T	H	E	R	I	N	G	

p. 140 Number teaser: Twenty-eight cookies are baked in each batch. The first tin fitted twenty-four cookies, and the second fits thirty-six.

p. 140 Deductions: Chris learns Norwegian on Mondays, Ali learns Spanish on Wednesdays, and Brian learns Japanese on Fridays.

Session 16

p. 141 Reflections: C

p. 141 Hidden words:

1 CHILE: I didn't eat lun**ch; I le**ft the house too early.

2 ITALY: Did you spot that cat-like animal? Was **it a ly**nx?

3 PANAMA: I find popping bubble wra**p an ama**zing stressbuster.

p. 142 Dominoes:

1	4	4	2	3	2
0	4	0	3	3	1
0	4	1	1	4	1
2	1	4	0	2	2
3	0	0	3	3	2

Session 17

p. 143 Shape count: twenty-four rectangles

p. 143 Start and end: R (RIVER, RAZOR, REACTOR, RANCOUR)

p. 144 Futoshiki:

4	1	3 > 2	6	5
1	6	2	5	3 < 4
2 < 4	5	3	1	6
3	5	1	6	4	2
5	3	6	4	2	1
6	2	4	1	5	3

Session 18

p. 145 Top-down view: B

p. 146 Word circle: The word that includes all the letters is tractor. Other words to find include act, actor, arc, art, car, carrot, cart, cat, coat, oar, oat, orca, rat, roar, taco, tact, tar, taro, tart, tat, and tract.

p. 146 Jigdoku:

E	C	A	D	F	B
A	B	D	F	E	C
B	D	E	C	A	F
F	A	C	E	B	D
C	E	F	B	D	A
D	F	B	A	C	E

Session 19

p. 147 Kakuro:

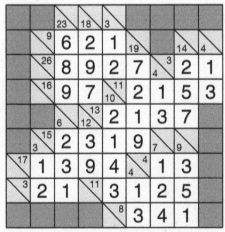

p. 148 Word ladder: one possible solution is NEXT → NEAT → PEAT → PEAK → PECK → PICK

p. 148 Tracing paper: D

Session 20

p. 149 Wordsearch:

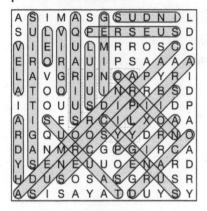

p. 150 Shapelink:

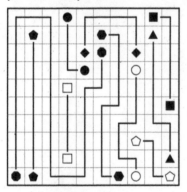

p. 151 Slitherlink:

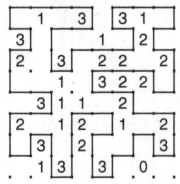

Session 21

p. 152 Sudoku:

4	8	3	9	6	7	5	2	1
9	7	2	1	8	5	4	6	3
1	6	5	2	4	3	9	8	7
7	4	6	5	2	1	8	3	9
5	2	8	4	3	9	7	1	6
3	1	9	8	7	6	2	4	5
6	5	4	3	9	8	1	7	2
8	3	1	7	5	2	6	9	4
2	9	7	6	1	4	3	5	8

p. 153 Touchy:

A	G	D	E	C	F	B
E	B	A	F	D	G	C
F	D	G	C	B	A	E
B	C	E	A	F	D	G
D	F	B	G	E	C	A
G	E	C	D	A	B	F
C	A	F	B	G	E	D

p. 154 Train tracks:

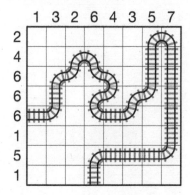

Level 3: Buckle-up puzzles

Session 22

p. 177 Building blocks: A

p. 177 Add a word: PICK (PICKUP, PICKAXE, PICKLED, PICKPOCKET)

p. 178 Age puzzle: Hamina is twenty-five, Ivy is seventeen, James is twenty-one, and Kai is twenty.

p. 178 Brainteaser: twice. The jeweller could split the gems into three piles of three gems and then weigh two of those piles against each other. If the scales balance, the fake is in the third pile. If they tip, the fake is in the lighter pile. The jeweller can then take two stones from the pile with the fake and weigh those. Either the scales will tip and the fake is therefore identified, or the scales will balance, in which case the gem that was not weighed is the fake.

Session 23

p. 181 Cube counting: thirty-four cubes

p. 182 Anagrams: TUNIS, RABAT, CAIRO, NAIROBI, KAMPALA, KINSHASA, KHARTOUM, MOGADISHU

p. 183 Number chains: 62, 50, 85, 54

p. 184 Calcudoku:

⁴⁻ 7	⁷⁰ˣ 5	1	¹²ˣ 4	3	⁴⁸ˣ 6	2
3	7	²¹⁰ˣ 6	5	³⁺ 2	1	4
2	1	7	²⁴ˣ 6	4	¹²ˣ 3	⁸⁺ 5
¹⁻ 6	⁵⁺ 2	¹⁻ 5	7	1	4	3
5	3	³⁻ 4	1	¹²⁶ˣ 6	²⁶⁺ 2	7
¹⁻ 1	⁶⁺ 4	2	3	7	5	⁶÷ 6
4	6	¹⁻ 3	2	5	7	1

Session 24

p. 187 Fold and punch: B

p. 187 Changed sets: birds (RAVEN, PETREL, ROBIN, SWAN, STARLING)

p. 188 Number darts: $33 = 9 + 20 + 4$; $51 = 25 + 8 + 18$; $59 = 11 + 35 + 13$

p. 188 Complete the series: D (At each stage the line with a dot rotates anti-clockwise by 45 degrees around the centre of the box. Conversely, the collection of other lines in the box rotates as a group clockwise by 90 degrees around the corners of the box, and an extra diagonal line is added to that set of lines.)

Session 25

p. 189 Hidden image: A

p. 189 Connected clues: fish (mullet, perch, sole, bass, fluke)

p. 190 Number pyramid:

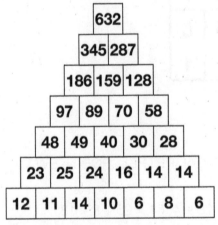

p. 191 Crack the code: b: NVEL (N = black dots; B = white dots; V = two dots; C = three dots; S = dots in bottom-left corner and oval centred; E = dots in top-right corner and oval to the left; P = white oval; L = grey oval)

Session 26

p. 192 Maze:

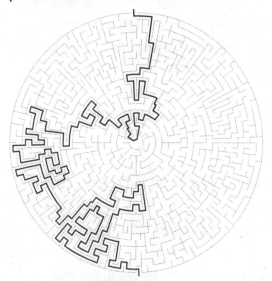

p. 193 Crossword:

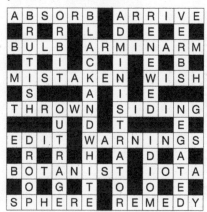

A	B	S	O	R	B		A	R	R	I	V	E
	R		R		L		D		E		E	
B	U	L	B		A	R	M	I	N	A	R	M
	T		I		C		I		E		B	
M	I	S	T	A	K	E	N		W	I	S	H
	S			A			I		E			
T	H	R	O	W	N		S	I	D	I	N	G
			U		D		T				E	
E	D	I	T		W	A	R	N	I	N	G	S
	R		R		H		A		D		A	
B	O	T	A	N	I	S	T		I	O	T	A
	O		G		T		O		O		E	
S	P	H	E	R	E		R	E	M	E	D	Y

p. 194 Number teaser: turn over both hourglasses at the same time. When the four-minute hourglass runs out, the chef should then put the biscuits in the oven. When the seven-minute hourglass also runs out – which will therefore be after a further three minutes – they should then turn the seven-minute hourglass over again. Once all the sand has run through it, ten minutes will have elapsed and the biscuits can be removed from the oven.

p. 194 Deductions: Sunita has a red door with a shell-shaped knocker, Verity has a green door with a claw-shaped knocker, Tegan has a blue door with a fox-shaped knocker, and Ursula has a white door with a leaf-shaped knocker.

Session 27

p. 195 Reflections: D

p. 195 Hidden words:

1   LIME: There's a phone cal**l I'm e**xpecting before lunch, so I might be hard to reach.

2   BANANA: Is 'thum**b' an ana**tomical term, or is there a more technical one?

3   LYCHEE: I usual**ly chee**r for the home team, but they played so badly today.

p. 196 Dominoes:

5	6	6	3	4	2	5	0
0	0	2	0	4	1	3	3
1	2	3	2	4	4	2	5
6	6	6	1	4	1	1	3
5	3	3	6	0	4	1	2
5	0	1	5	5	4	3	2
5	1	0	4	2	6	6	0

Session 28

p. 197 Shape count: thirty-eight rectangles

p. 197 Start and end: E (ELITE, ERASE, ELOPE, EAGLE)

p. 198 Futoshiki:

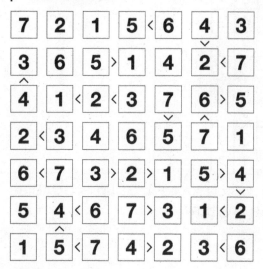

Session 29

p. 199 Top-down view: A

p. 200 Word circle: the word that includes all the letters is defiance. Other words to find include ace, aced, acid, acne, aid, aide, and, cad, cafe, can, cane, caned, dace, dance, deaf, dean, deface, face, faced, fad, fade, fain, fan, fancied, fiance, fiancee and idea.

p. 200 Jigdoku:

F	A	G	C	D	E	B
E	B	D	A	G	C	F
G	E	F	B	A	D	C
D	C	A	E	B	F	G
B	G	C	F	E	A	D
C	D	E	G	F	B	A
A	F	B	D	C	G	E

Session 30

p. 201 Kakuro:

	12	12				9	3
12	9	3	4		4 / 11	3	1
6	3	2	1	10 / 7	1	4	2
	11	7	3	1	9 / 12	7	2
		6 / 12	2	1	3		
	12 / 6	2	7	3	4	6	
	12 / 12	3	9	13	8	3	2 / 11
6	3	2	1		13	1	3	9
10	9	1			3	1	2

p. 202 Word ladder: one possible solution is GOLD → GOAD → ROAD → ROAR → SOAR → STAR

p. 202 Tracing paper: B

Session 31

p. 203 Wordsearch:

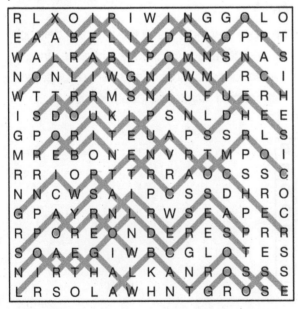

p. 204 Shapelink:

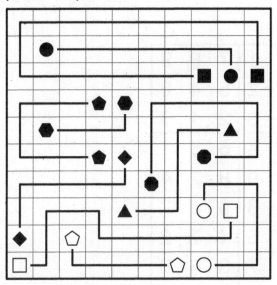

p. 205 Slitherlink:

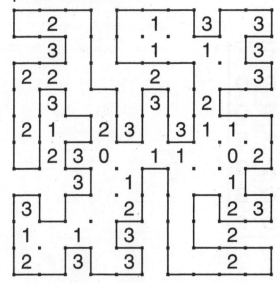

Session 32

p. 206 Sudoku:

3	6	2	5	4	1	7	8	9
1	9	8	3	7	2	5	4	6
4	5	7	9	8	6	2	1	3
9	8	3	7	2	4	6	5	1
6	7	5	1	3	9	8	2	4
2	1	4	6	5	8	9	3	7
8	3	6	4	9	5	1	7	2
5	4	9	2	1	7	3	6	8
7	2	1	8	6	3	4	9	5

p. 207 Touchy:

F	D	B	C	G	E	A
C	A	G	E	F	B	D
B	E	F	D	A	G	C
D	G	A	B	C	F	E
E	B	C	F	D	A	G
G	F	D	A	E	C	B
A	C	E	G	B	D	F

p. 208 Train tracks:

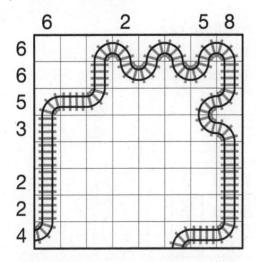

Level 4: Don't-give-up puzzles

Session 33

p. 213 Building blocks: D

p. 213 Add a word: HORSE (HORSEBACK, HORSEPOWER, HORSEPLAY, HORSESHOE)

p. 214 Age puzzle: Lucy is forty-two, Meg is fifty-six, Nora is thirty, and Omar is thirty-eight.

p. 214 Brainteaser: Emma. For Dave to play four games and lose them all, he must have played in the second, fourth, sixth, and eighth games, since we know that Emma lost the first one. If Emma lost the first game, Faisal must have won it, which began his winning streak. After the third game, we know that neither Dave nor Faisal wins again, so Emma must have won the fifth game.

Session 34

p. 217 Cube counting: twenty-five cubes

p. 218 Anagrams: BOSCH, TITIAN, RAPHAEL, HOLBEIN, DONATELLO, TINTORETTO, BOTTICELLI, MICHELANGELO

p. 219 Number chains: 619, 383, 185, 191

p. 220 Calcudoku:

2- **1**	2÷ **6**	**3**	6+ **2**	3- **4**	**7**	13+ **8**	**5**
3	48× **4**	**6**	**1**	**2**	240× **8**	**5**	11+ **7**
20× **5**	**2**	56× **7**	**8**	**1**	15× **3**	**6**	**4**
4	26+ **7**	**8**	540× **6**	**3**	**5**	56× **2**	**1**
8	**3**	2× **1**	**5**	**6**	**4**	**7**	6× **2**
1- **7**	25× **5**	**2**	19+ **4**	2- **8**	**6**	8× **1**	**3**
6	**1**	**5**	**3**	**7**	**2**	**4**	48× **8**
16× **2**	**8**	28× **4**	**7**	**5**	3÷ **1**	**3**	**6**

Session 35

p. 223 Fold and punch: C

p. 223 Changed sets: capital cities (PARIS, PRAGUE, ROME, TUNIS, BERN)

p. 224 Number darts: 42 = 23 + 16 + 3; 59 = 24 + 32 + 3; 82 = 10 + 38 + 34

p. 224 Complete the series: C (At each stage any thin circle becomes a thick circle, or if no thin circle is present then a new thin circle is added to the outside of the group in the centre. Also, the triangle rotates 90 degrees around the centre of the box, and then after moving and rotating it flips direction to point the opposite way.)

Session 36

p. 225 Hidden image: D

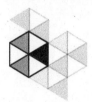

p. 225 Connected clues: lakes (Superior, Victoria, Bled, Crater, Reindeer)

p. 226 Number pyramid:

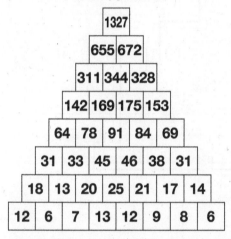

p. 227 Crack the code: d: RGJZ (R = grey star on top; T = white star on top; Y = grey star points down; G = grey star points up; J = white dots on bar; K = black dots on bar; A = vertical bar; Z = horizontal bar)

Session 37

p. 228 Maze:

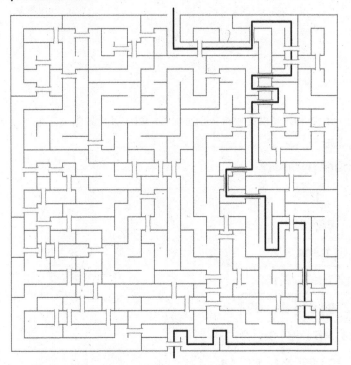

p. 229 Number teaser: one leaf.

pp. 230–231 Spiral crossword:

Inwards		Outwards	
1–6	BURSAR	**100–95**	DECIDE
7–11	ELEGY	**94–90**	TACIT
12–14	ORE	**89–85**	SALES
15–19	CIVIC	**84–82**	TIN
20–24	OLDER	**81–76**	UNLIKE
25–28	RATS	**75–71**	LADEN
29–31	RED	**70–66**	ANISE
32–36	LEGAL	**65–61**	PATHS
37–41	FUNGI	**60–58**	AWE
42–44	NAP	**57–54**	YEAH
45–50	MITTEN	**53–48**	PLANET
51–55	ALPHA	**47–41**	TIMPANI
56–62	EYEWASH	**40–38**	GNU
63–67	TAPES	**37–34**	FLAG
68–72	INANE	**33–29**	ELDER
73–76	DALE	**28–22**	STARRED
77–80	KILN	**21–18**	LOCI
81–85	UNITS	**17–11**	VICEROY
86–96	ELASTICATED	**10–8**	GEL
97–100	ICED	**7–4**	ERAS
		3–1	RUB

p. 232 Deductions: There are eight pink tulips, four orange roses and six yellow gerberas.

Session 38

p. 233 Reflections: B

p. 233 Hidden words:

1 ALPACA: Some hairdressers give the sc**alp a ca**reful massage when washing hair.

2 ARMADILLO: Please don't make the vic**ar mad, I'll o**nly have to apologise later.

3 PORCUPINE: Do you have a spare sugar lum**p, or cup? I ne**ed two of everything for a tea party.

p. 234 Dominoes:

1	3	6	1	5	2	0	4
2	6	4	5	3	3	5	3
2	6	1	1	5	0	5	4
1	4	2	4	4	6	1	1
0	0	6	0	3	2	2	5
3	2	5	1	0	6	0	3
3	6	2	6	0	4	4	5

Session 39

p. 235 Shape count: thirty-three rectangles

p. 235 Start and end: W (WITHDRAW, WORKFLOW, WINNOW, WIDOW)

p. 236 Futoshiki:

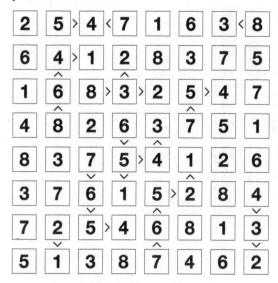

Session 40

p. 237 Top-down view: C

p. 238 Word circle: the word that includes all the letters is posterity. Other words to find include espy, opt, opts, osprey, per, pert, peso, pest, pesto, pet, pets, petty, pie, pier, piers, pies, piety, pis, pit, pits, pity, poet, poetry, poets, poi, poise, pore, pores, port, ports, pose, poser, posit, post, poster, posy, pot, pots, potter, potters, pottery, potties, potty, presto, pretty, prey, preys, pries, priest, prise, pro, pros, prose, protest, pry, pyre, pyres, pyrite, pyrites, rip, ripe, ripes, ripest, riposte, rips, rope, ropes, sip, sop, spire, spit, spite, spore, sport, sporty, spot, spotter, spottier, spotty, sprit, sprite, spry, spy, step, stop, strep, strip, stripe, strop, tip, tips, tipster, tipsy, tiptoe, tiptoes, top, tops, trip, tripe, tripos, trips, trope, tropes, type, types, typist, yip and yips.

p. 238 Jigdoku:

H	G	B	A	C	F	D	E
F	D	A	E	G	C	B	H
C	E	D	H	F	B	G	A
B	H	C	F	D	E	A	G
G	A	E	D	B	H	F	C
E	F	G	B	H	A	C	D
A	C	F	G	E	D	H	B
D	B	H	C	A	G	E	F

Session 41

p. 239 Kakuro:

				16	21	7	
	6	15	21 / 12	9	8	4	
4	1	3	19 / 17	2	7	9	1
18	5	4	8	1	6 / 13	4	2
	22	8	9	3	2	13	23
		15	30 / 11	6	7	8	9	4
	16	9	7	15 / 5	3	5	6	1
	10	4	3	2	1	11	8	3
	6	2	1	3			

p. 240 Word ladder: one possible solution is START → STARE → SHARE → SHORE → CHORE → CHOSE → CLOSE

p. 240 Tracing paper: C

Session 42

p. 241 Wordsearch:

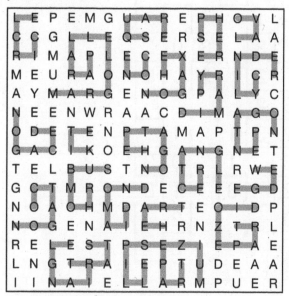

p. 242 Shapelink:

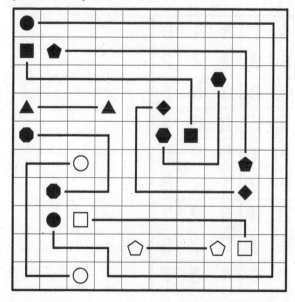

p. 243 Slitherlink:

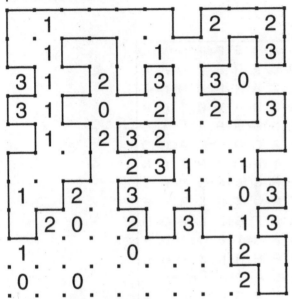

Session 43

p. 244 Sudoku:

6	5	3	2	4	7	8	1	9
9	8	1	5	6	3	7	4	2
7	4	2	1	9	8	3	6	5
3	1	7	9	5	6	2	8	4
4	2	8	3	7	1	5	9	6
5	6	9	4	8	2	1	7	3
8	9	5	7	3	4	6	2	1
2	7	4	6	1	5	9	3	8
1	3	6	8	2	9	4	5	7

p. 245 Touchy:

F	E	G	H	B	D	A	C
D	C	F	A	G	E	B	H
A	B	E	C	H	F	D	G
C	G	D	B	E	A	H	F
B	H	A	F	D	G	C	E
G	D	B	E	C	H	F	A
H	A	C	G	F	B	E	D
E	F	H	D	A	C	G	B

p. 246 Train tracks:

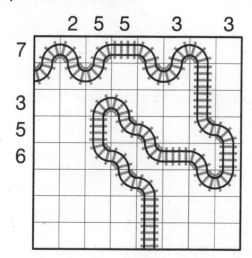

Acknowledgements

One of the joys of writing is connecting with new researchers and clinicians. I am particularly grateful to the following people, who kindly read and improved some or all of this book: Prof Joy Bhattacharya (Department of Psychology, Goldsmiths University of London), Dr Dorina Cadar (Centre for Dementia Studies, Brighton and Sussex Medical School), Dr Claire Durrant (UK Dementia Research Institute Emerging Leader, University of Edinburgh), Reinhard Guss (Consultant Clinical Psychologist, Oxleas NHS Foundation Trust), Dr Gemma Lace (Biomedical Research Centre, University of Salford), Prof Gill Livingston (Professor of Psychiatry of Older People, University College London), Dr Lan Nguyen (School of Applied Psychology, Griffith University), Emma Twyning (Centre for Ageing Better), and Dr Aideen Young (Centre for Ageing Better). Any errors that remain are mine alone.

Variously present at the conception, gestation, and delivery of *Mind Games* were agent Adam Gauntlett of Peters Fraser + Dunlop, and Zennor Compton and Callum Crute at Penguin Random House. Also at PRH, Laurie Ip Fung Chun and Anna Cowling, as well as freelancers Odhran O'Donoghue, Dan Prescott and Jonathan Wadman, edited, checked, designed, proofread, and produced with skill and attention. At Alzheimer's Society, huge thanks go to Georgie Davies, Angharad Jones,

James Baulk, and Tatjana Trposka. The book and my mental health are so much better for all these people's encouragement, wisdom and kindness.

Finally, my deepest gratitude goes to my family, Sarah and the boys – always and for everything. Thank you.

Further reading

Try the following if you want to know more about some of the topics in *Mind Games*.

Cobb, M. *The Idea of the Brain: A History.* London: Profile Books, 2021.

Doidge, N. *The Brain That Changes Itself: Stories of Personal Triumph from the Frontiers of Brain Science.* New York, NY: Penguin, 2007.

Eagleman, D. *The Brain: The Story of You.* Edinburgh: Canongate Books, 2015.

Eagleman, D. *Livewired: The Inside Story of the Ever-Changing Brain.* Edinburgh: Canongate Books, 2021.

Fernyhough, C. *Pieces of Light: The New Science of Memory.* London: Profile Books, 2012.

Goodwin, G. *Supercharge Your Brain: How to Maintain a Healthy Brain Throughout Your Life.* London: Penguin, 2021.

Jacobs, A J, and Pliska, G. *The Puzzler: One Man's Quest to Solve the Most Baffling Puzzles Ever, from Crosswords to Jigsaws to the Meaning of Life.* New York, NY: Crown, 2022.

Kandel, E. *In Search of Memory: The Emergence of a New Science of Mind*. New York, NY: W W Norton, 2006.

Kuhn, G. *Experiencing the Impossible: The Science of Magic*. Cambridge, MA: MIT Press, 2019.

Lehrer, J. *Proust Was a Neuroscientist*. Edinburgh: Canongate Books, 2012.

Levitin, D J. *The Changing Mind: A Neuroscientist's Guide to Ageing Well*. London: Penguin Life, 2021.

Shaw, J. *The Memory Illusion: Remembering, Forgetting, and the Science of False Memory*. London: Random House, 2016.

Steele, A. *Ageless: The New Science of Getting Older Without Getting Old*. London: Bloomsbury, 2020.

Walker, M. *Why We Sleep: The New Science of Sleep and Dreams*. London: Penguin, 2018.